PRAISE FOR

LIVING WITHOUT DIETING

"LIVING WITHOUT DIETING is not a traditional diet book, offering a miracle cure or a quick fix. It's more of a workbook, designed to help readers come to grips with the underlying forces that may cause them to overeat or underexercise....One of the best features: self-evaluations that can help the reader maintain motivation. I'm going to recommend this to my clients."

— Cathie Pfarr, *USA Today*

"A good book....LIVING WITHOUT DIETING gets this dietitian's vote."

— Gail A. Levey, R.D., *Parade* magazine

"Of the many books written by researchers at weight-loss clinics, LIVING WITHOUT DIETING is among the best."

— *Working Woman*

"The authors are to be commended for translating what experts know into what those concerned about weight should know."

— David Garner, Ph.D., professor, Department of Psychiatry, Michigan State University

"Presents a realistic and clear way to deal with obesity in a society obsessed with thinness."

— *Calorie Control Commentary*

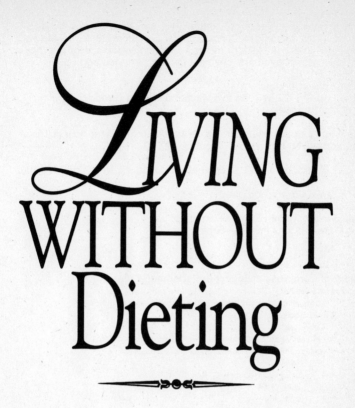

LIVING WITHOUT Dieting

JOHN P. FOREYT, Ph.D.

AND

G. KEN GOODRICK, Ph.D.

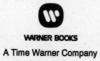

WARNER BOOKS

A Time Warner Company

Warner Books Edition
Copyright © 1992 by John P. Foreyt and G. Ken Goodrick
All rights reserved.

This Warner Books edition is published by arrangement with Harrison Publishing, P.O. Box 540515, Houston, TX 77254-0515

Warner Books, Inc., 1271 Avenue of the Americas, New York, NY 10020

W A Time Warner Company

Printed in the United States of America
First Warner Books Printing: September 1994
10 9 8 7 6 5 4 3 2 1

Library of Congress Cataloging-in-Publication Data
  Foreyt, John Paul.
      Living without dieting / John P. Foreyt and G. Ken Goodrick.--
  Warner Books ed.
        p.   cm.
      Originally published: Houston, Tex. : Harrison Pub., c1992.
      Includes bibliographical references and index.
      ISBN 0-446-38269-8 :
      1. Reducing. I. Goodrick, G. Ken. II. Title.
  RM222.2.F674   1994
  613.2'5--dc20   93-46709
                                                              CIP

Cover design by Diane Luger
Cover photograph by Nancy Pulibniak
Aria Golo silverware by Christofle
Tableware by Lenox China & Crystal

ACKNOWLEDGMENTS

This book represents the efforts of two psychologist/researchers who have a combined 35 years experience in studying weight management problems. Our ideas come from many researchers and pioneers, some of whom are referenced in this book. They also come from individuals who have sought help and who have participated as subjects in various research projects. We recognize our debt and express our gratitude to all of them.

The treatment of weight problems involves many disciplines. We especially wish to thank the following individuals who have supported our efforts on this book. From the field of psychology: Jennifer H. Cousins, Ph.D., Carol B. Hailes, Ph.D., Gayle D. Pitcher, Ph.D., and David M. Garner, Ph.D. From medicine: C. Wayne Callaway, M.D. and Simon P. Petrides, M.B., B.S., D.O., M.R.O., Dip. Sports Med. From dietetics: Patricia W. Pace, M.S., R.D., Rebecca S. Reeves, M.P.H., R.D., Adele Huls, R.D., Rosemary Gonzalez, M.S., R.D., and Hortencia Mendoza-Martinez, M.P.H., R.D. From the specialty of psychotherapy of eating disorders: Donna R. Pittman, C.S.W.-A.C.P., and Retta Parker, R.N., C.E.D.T. From exercise science: A. S. 'Tony' Jackson, P.E.D. Valuable insights have also been obtained from the nursing profession: Barbara Sheldon Czerwinski, M.S.N., R.N., Jennifer Scott Cooper, M.S., R.N., and Mary Pat Bolton, R.D., L.D.

Finally, a special thanks to our literary production manager, Alan H. Brown, who has helped with everything from word processing tips to international copyrighting.

ABOUT THE AUTHORS

John P. Foreyt, Ph.D., received his training at the University of Wisconsin, Florida State University and the University of Southern California Medical Center. He is currently Professor, Department of Medicine, Baylor College of Medicine and Director of the Nutrition Research Clinic. Dr. Foreyt has been awarded research grants from the National Institutes of Health and other organizations in the areas of diet modification, cardiovascular risk reduction, eating disorders and obesity. He has published 13 books and over 120 papers in scientific journals.

G. Ken Goodrick, Ph.D., CEAP, has been researching and treating obesity for over a decade. A former NASA engineer, he received his psychological training at the University of Houston and Baylor College of Medicine. He is currently Assistant Professor of Medicine at Baylor College of Medicine, where his work at the Nutrition Research Clinic involves treatment of obesity and eating/exercise disorders.

TABLE OF CONTENTS

Preface...ix

The Frustrated Dieter's Quiz...............................xi

1. New Ways of Thinking..................................1

2. Is Obesity Hereditary?.................................15

3. The Mind Versus Body Problem.................25

4. Lookism and the Obese Self........................43

5. Social Support...63

6. Becoming an Exercise Enthusiast...............81

7. How to Become a Low-Fat Eater..............109

8. The Plan...127

Appendix A: Getting Professional Help........151

Appendix B: Resources..................................161

Appendix C: References.................................171

Appendix D: Self-Evaluation.........................181

Appendix E: Fat Grams Per Serving..............197

Index..203

PREFACE

Over $32 billion is spent each year on weight control efforts. Most people receiving treatment lose weight, but then many gain it all back and perhaps even more. Continued attempts to lose weight often lead to the yo-yo phenomenon of weight fluctuation. Yo-yo weight fluctuation is frustrating and depressing. It may also increase the risk of cardiovascular disease. The bottom line is this: a lot of money is being spent, and the ultimate result for many people may be injury to mental and physical health.

The accepted treatments for obesity seem, for many individuals, to do more harm than good.[1] In order to help rectify this situation, we have, along with our colleagues in ethics and health policy, published a series of papers in scientific journals about weight management.[2-6] This book presents our recommendations to the public based on these papers.

The treatment program we recommend will help overweight individuals achieve optimal physical and mental health. It requires changes in lifestyle, attitude and relationships with others. With some courage, individuals can achieve a satisfactory weight management outcome. In the process, they will also escape from their obese self: the self that has kept them trapped in frustration and disappointment.

This book is designed to help individuals who fail in trying to manage their weight. It should benefit those who have difficulty controlling their consumption of fatty foods, and those who have trouble sticking to an exercise program. Those individuals who vomit, or use laxatives or diuretics regularly to control their weight may also be helped by this book, but they must first consult with an eating disorders therapist and a physician. Those who have serious depression or excessive stress are advised to see a psychologist before beginning.

This book outlines a lifetime program. Individuals should read it carefully all the way through before starting the program and keep it handy for reference. Favorite parts should be read frequently to keep up motivation.

Be sure to complete the Awareness Exercises by writing in this book. The Awareness Exercises ask the same kinds of questions a therapist might ask. They are designed to clarify thinking by getting thoughts out on paper. This will make the book a personal record for later reference.

Remember, *Living Without Dieting* helps develop a lifetime program. Have a relaxed attitude. Take things slowly. Think in terms of months or years. Be good to yourself.

Individuals should get the approval of their physician before beginning this program. This is obvious if they have any medical conditions. They may also have some hidden disorder about which they are unaware. Only a physician can be responsible for taking care of physical conditions, and ensuring that a program is safe.

JPF
GKG

THE FRUSTRATED DIETER'S QUIZ

Circle the statements which are true:

1. I am frustrated about my inability to stick to a diet.

2. I feel I have less self-control than most dieters.

3. Most of the times I try to lose weight, I lose control and go off my diet.

4. When I try to develop a habit of regular exercise, something always interferes and I stop.

5. Exercise seems to be an ordeal to me.

6. I often feel tired during the day.

7. My weight has gone up and down several times as I go on and off diets.

8. My body seems to be getting thicker in the middle over the years.

9. My weight seems to be increasing over the years.

10. I find myself thinking about food more than I should.

11. I find myself thinking about my weight problem all through the day.

12. I feel there is probably no hope for my weight problem.

13. I eat fattening foods only when no one can see me.

14. Sometimes I lose control and really binge on food.

15. I use food to make myself feel better when I am angry, nervous, or depressed.

16. Some people reject me as a friend because I am too heavy.

17. My social life is limited because of my weight.

18. My sex life is limited because of my weight.

19. Other people think I am unattractive because of my weight.

20. I put a lot of effort into wearing clothes which tend to cover up my weight problem.

21. I have no one to blame but myself for my weight problem.

22. I feel inadequate as a person because I know that I need therapy to really succeed in weight control.

23. Sometimes I feel that I deserve to get less out of life because I don't have enough willpower to control my weight.

Compare the statements that you found to be true with the following areas:

Dieting self-control: statements 1,2,3

Many overweight people have tried and failed at dieting. It leads to frustration and feeling out of control. But there are physiological and psychological reasons why you shouldn't blame yourself for dieting failure. More importantly, trying to eat too little on a diet may make your problem only worse. Read Chapters 1,2,3 and 7.

Exercise self-control: statements 4,5,6

If other things seem to interfere with your exercise, you may need help making exercise a priority in your life. Do you feel exercise is an ordeal? Do you feel tired much of the time? Read Chapter 6.

Health status and overweight: statements 7,8,9

Weight fluctuation due to repeated dieting may be harmful to your health. There is also an increased risk for disease if your body fat seems to be shifting to your middle rather than to your thighs. If your weight keeps increasing, you may increase your risk of back trouble, arthritis pain and other disorders. Read Chapter 2.

Disturbing thoughts: statements 10,11,12

After repeated failures to manage weight, many people end up obsessed about food and their weight problem; these concerns take priority over other matters, even family and job. Along with these thoughts is an overriding feeling of despair. Read Chapters 3,4 and 5.

Abnormal eating episodes: statements 13,14,15

Secretive eating, binge eating and using food to make yourself feel better are signs of a possible disturbed relationship with food. Shame leads to secrecy about eating; this needs to be addressed in small groups where individuals can share their experiences and realize that they should not be ashamed of a problem which is really caused by misinformation about dieting and intense social pressure to be thin.

Binge eating may be caused by dieting; it is like gasping uncontrollably for air after trying to breathe very shallowly for a long time. If you have dieted a lot, your body may increase its craving for food. This may make eating especially enjoyable, so that eating becomes a way to relieve negative emotions. Read Chapters 1,2,3 and 4.

Social isolation: statements 16,17,18

Due to discrimination against overweight people and the feelings of shame related to overweight and abnormal eating, many overweight individuals become socially isolated. Close relationships are vital to happiness. Learning to establish relationships begins in small groups with other individuals who have similar problems. Read Chapter 5.

Self-consciousness: statements 19,20

Many people in our society are overly concerned about their appearance; overweight people may have a greater concern because of the value of thinness in our culture. Read Chapter 4.

Self-blame: statements 21,22,23

 Many overweight people blame themselves for their inability to manage their weight. Their lack of control is due largely to the fact that for most people dieting is not only an ineffective method for weight management but may actually make the problem worse. Read Chapters 1 and 3.

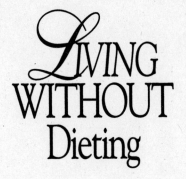

LIVING
WITHOUT
Dieting

1

NEW WAYS OF THINKING

———

Being overweight is a problem millions of Americans have. Over 32 billion dollars is spent each year in this country on attempts to lose unattractive pounds. Researchers have been looking for a *cure* since research began. Since 1986, over 600 papers have been published in scientific journals on the treatment of obesity. And yet, despite these heroic efforts, despite this diet and that exercise program, despite this formula or that drug, Americans are fatter than ever before in history.

It appears that the solution to the obesity problem is a mystery. In this book we explore why people become overweight and why they don't maintain weight losses. We explain why many overweight people are tricked into becoming their own worst enemy in the battle of the bulge. We present an alternate way of looking at the obesity problem. It is our hope that this book can help free many from the pain of obesity.

In order to solve the mystery of obesity, we use several metaphors which are designed to help develop new ways of thinking about weight problems. Through these metaphors, we describe how obesity is related to:

- Bearded tits (rare birds) in a zoo
- Breath holding
- A boulder in a stream
- A Chinese finger puzzle
- A forest ranger's bathroom habits

The Bearded Tit Mystery[1]

At a major zoological garden in Europe, two rare bearded tits were held captive for viewing by humans. These birds were so rare that the ornithologists made every effort to keep the birds healthy and to help them reproduce. The birds had the finest cage, large enough for good flying. The food was grown especially for the birds in a special garden stocked with plants from their native land. Temperature and humidity were precisely controlled. One-way mirrors were used so that the birds couldn't see the human observers or be disturbed by the noise of children. All needed nesting materials were furnished.

The birds mated successfully, producing fertile eggs, and the hen dutifully kept the eggs warm. The hatchlings emerged from the eggs looking quite healthy. The young birds would beg for food as soon as they emerged, and the parents would provide them with an ample supply of regurgitated food. But on the third or fourth day, the parents would pick up the chicks, and unceremoniously drop them out of the nest, onto the ground. Left uncared for, they perished.

This phenomenon recurred several times with new sets of chicks. The keepers were mystified. Why did these birds regularly practice infanticide even when their surroundings duplicated those found in their native habitat? It seemed the birds were programmed to kill their offspring. Obviously, this could not be an instinctive behavior, or this species of bird would have been wiped out in the first generation. But it turned out to be related to an instinctive behavior.

Birds do many things on the basis of instinct. We are constantly amazed by some of the incredibly complex behavior patterns of birds. Mating dances and fancy feather displays, nest building, egg sitting and regurgitation to feed the young are all *programmed* through genetic transmission. This automatic programming almost always helps the species to survive.

So why then did the bearded tits dump their newborns? The answer lies in a species adaptation to maintain hygiene and to avoid disease. It is obvious that a dead chick left in the nest will gather flies and disease. We would not question a parent bird discarding a dead chick. The key to the problem can be found by comparing the behavior of the young birds at the zoo with their cousins in the wild.

In their natural habitat, adult birds stake out territory around their nest, which they protect from incursion by other birds of the same species. This ensures them of a food supply. But, over time, the number of birds grows until the available territory for each bird, or bird pair, shrinks to the point where the food supply becomes limited. The task of mustering up enough bugs for the family takes all day, and the supply is just enough to survive.

Under these conditions, the chicks are in a state of constant hunger, which they indicate with upturned heads and open beaks. The adult birds are instinctively programmed to regurgitate food into these squawking gullets. Unfortunately for their zoo-born counterparts, the food supply set up by the ornithologists was not only the finest available but also abundant in quantity. So abundant that the parents soon were able to satisfy the young chicks' appetite. The youngsters took long naps. The naps lasted so long that the adults' instinctive drive to rid the nest of dead chicks took

3

over, and out they went. To solve this problem the zookeepers had only to limit the food supply to these birds. This kept the chicks hungry, active and alive.

This is an example of what happens when there is a mismatch between the needs of an animal and the food supply offered by the environment. For most species, the problem is always undersupply of food. Modern human society has developed to the point where the food supply for humans in the industrialized nations is not only overly adequate in quantity but is also richer in fat than needed for normal functioning. We are programmed to eat, and to crave high-energy (high-calorie) foods. This is an instinctive adaptation for humans which evolved before food was plentiful.

The lesson of the birds for overweight humans is that the problem may in part be due to a mismatch between the food environment and human nutritional needs. Fast-food restaurants are conveniently located everywhere. Humans are *instinctively programmed* to eat high-fat foods even though most individuals know the consequences. Many overweight people feel *dumped* out of the nest of society because they are too fat. Perhaps we all need a zookeeper to regulate our food supply.

Breath Holding

How long can individuals hold their breath? No one can stop breathing indefinitely. Even the mystics of the East who seem able to go without breathing for long periods must eventually continue breathing. We are programmed by our nervous system to breathe automatically. Although we can stop breathing temporarily, after a while our lower nervous system takes over, and we gasp for fresh air, despite our *will* to hold our breath longer.

Now suppose someone was told that to be a worthwhile person she had to be able to hold her breath for five minutes. Suppose everyone told her that. Suppose she actually believed it was true. She would probably try to achieve a 5-minute non-breathing period. Why? Because as social beings, we want and need to be loved and to feel worthwhile.

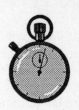

But of course this is a ridiculous example since everyone knows that for almost everyone it is impossible to stop breathing for five minutes. If she tried to do it and failed, no one would blame her, since everyone recognizes that we cannot have complete control over our breathing function.

However, suppose everyone told her that in order to be a worthwhile person, she had to restrict her eating until she lost a lot of weight? Suppose she tried, and lost many pounds, but then went back to her old eating habits and regained the lost weight? Would people blame her then? Would she blame herself?

Our research shows that 90 percent of overweight people blame themselves for failure to keep off weight lost through dieting. And 90 percent of all persons who try to lose weight by dieting ultimately fail and regain. This adds up to a lot of failure and self-blame.

We feel that losing weight by dieting is not unlike breath holding. The body will take over control after a while, and it will cause breathing and eating even if the mind doesn't want to. After breath holding, a normal person will inhale a vast quantity of air to make up for the oxygen deficit. After a prolonged diet, the body will take in a large number of calories to make up for caloric deprivation.

The question for the reader is: Should individuals continue to blame themselves for having a perfectly natural bodily reaction to dieting? We talk more about the psychology of dieting and how it often leads to eating disorders in Chapter Three.

A Boulder in the Stream

The story is told of an impulsive young man who wanted to remove a large boulder from the middle of a stream so that his fishing boat could pass by. He was so impetuous that he ran into the stream and started heaving his body against the rock. It would not budge. The man grasped recklessly at the rock with his bare hands, cutting his hands and wrists. The rock moved only slightly. So intense became this man's passion to move the stone that he did not notice his increasing loss of blood. Soon his fatigue and loss of blood caused him to faint. He fell face down in the water and drowned. Many years later, the stream wore down the boulder into a few pebbles.

The lesson here is that sometimes a gradual approach is needed. If a woman gained 50 pounds of excess fat over ten years, she shouldn't push herself trying to lose it in two months. There are two reasons for this. First, it can be painful and dangerous to lose weight too fast. Second, quick losses may set up the body to conserve energy so that regain is likely, and she would end up worse off than ever.

We believe in gradual weight loss. Our advertisements might well proclaim:

Lose 50 pounds in two years!

Would this get you excited? In Chapter Three we discuss the psychology of gradualism, which we feel is one of the keys to ultimate success.

A Chinese Finger Puzzle

We often tell our patients that weight loss is like getting out of a Chinese finger puzzle. If you pull hard to try to get out fast, you become more firmly caught. The correct approach is a gradual easing and twisting motion. In this book, we present several new *twists* to the weight-loss game.

A Forest Ranger's Bathroom Habits

Years ago, before earth satellites and other technologies, men were sent to spend long periods sitting on top of tall observation towers to spot forest fires. The lore of this profession has it that new observers would go through some interesting changes during their first stint. A new man would shave daily, bathe almost daily, wear reasonably clean clothes, and obey most of the rules set up for his vocation.

One rule was that urination would take place in the outhouse designed for that purpose. Every few hours, the observer would climb down the tower, walk over to the outhouse, and relieve himself. He would then climb up the tower and resume his observations.

After some days of this, it occurred to these men that as long as they were observant and reported in regularly by radio to headquarters, they could just about do as they pleased, since no one was watching them. So these men would become unkempt. Their quarters would become disarrayed. Clothes were washed only when they became unbearable. Dishes were washed only when needed. They became mountain men. And they urinated right off the top of the tower, downwind.

But if they were to be visited, a return to the norms of civility came about posthaste. The point is, we do a lot of things because of social scrutiny: people are watching. We want to be accepted as normal, worthwhile people. We are afraid of rejection if we do not conform. Most of us conform.

How does this apply to the plight of the obese? This is the Great Obesity Paradox. It goes something like this:

Overweight people feel social pressure to be thin. They feel discriminated against and ostracized. This can lead to social isolation and private eating behavior, as well as depression with low self-esteem, leading to reduced self-control. Isolation and privacy serve to make the problem worse. Perceived social pressure to be thin is thus both the motivation for weight loss as well as an impediment to the self-control needed to achieve it.

The answer to controlling eating and exercise behaviors may lie in employing a different kind of social scrutiny. Since perceived social scrutiny from the general public can be a negative and destructive force (see Chapter Four), there is a need for the overweight to get social scrutiny from a new source. That new source is understanding peers, who have weight problems themselves. More on this in Chapter Five.

To return to the forest observer analogy, if someone were watching him, he would be less likely to deviate from norms of acceptable social behavior. But in the case of obesity, it is not usually a case of the obese person failing to eat and exercise appropriately just because no one is *watching*. It is partly that, but mostly it is because the weight-loss behaviors which are socially acceptable (dieting) are not effective for losing weight and maintaining that loss.

If current weight-loss strategies are effective, then why don't more overweight people succeed? We certainly cannot fault their motivation, since the pain of obesity leads to heroic, if not successful, efforts. We feel that it is a combination of method and the perceived social pressure to be thin which combine to make most people's struggles with weight futile.

The problem of method is that most people try to lose weight too fast, with too great a reliance on dietary restriction and too little emphasis on exercise. The problem with use of social pressure is that it is usually thought of as a negative force. These two problems are linked together by the one big problem: vanity. Our vanity compels us to lose weight too quickly. Our vanity views rejection by the Society of the Thin as a motivating force. Fast weight loss driven by negative emotions is doomed to failure. In the case of obesity, one can indeed be one's worst enemy. More on this in Chapter Four.

We hope to explain the psychology of successful weight management in the following chapters. We hope to help the overweight to stop punishing themselves for failure to lose weight and keep it off. We hope to show how to break through the social isolation and self-hatred that obesity may have caused.

We hope to demonstrate that by changing ideas about what works, and by turning negative emotions about social rejection into positive emotions of social support, that any overweight person can break free of the obesity trap, and achieve a healthy weight.

THE BOTTOM LINE:

- Like the birds in the zoo, our food environment is too fatty and plentiful.
- Like breath holding, dieting is against nature; nature will always win.
- A gradual approach is needed, even if a person is desperate to lose weight.
- Peer social support is needed; pressure from society is best ignored.

Awareness Exercises

1. Make a list of all the places (supermarkets, restaurants) where you can easily obtain high-fat foods:

    _____

    _____

    _____

    _____

    Compare the availability of high-fat foods now with the availability to pioneer women in 1850.

2. Describe how desperate you have felt to lose weight at various times in your life:

    _____

    _____

    _____

    _____

    Now relax and realize that it is time to let go of your feelings of desperation. These feelings cause anxiety and may reduce eating control. They also may cause you to try to lose weight too fast.

3.   About how many times have you tried to lose weight by
      dieting?

      _____

      *Have you finally realized that dieting is doomed to
      failure? Are you ready to try a different way?*

4.   How many times have you succeeded in keeping a lot of
      weight off for a long time?

      _____

      *If your diet fails, your weight fluctuates. This may be
      bad for health as well as self-esteem.*

5.   Describe your emotions when you have just begun a
      weight-loss diet:

      _____

      _____

      _____

      _____

      *Going on a diet is like taking a drug. It gives you a brief
      "high" because you lose weight and feel more energy for a
      short period of time. But over the long haul, it is harmful.*

6. Describe your emotions when you feel you have failed to keep off lost weight:

_____

_____

_____

_____

If you blame yourself for failing to stick to a diet, you are adding insult to injury. Your self-esteem may already be injured because of the social stigma against obesity. It is very painful to have low self-esteem and to think of yourself as failing again.

7. Describe how you have felt discriminated against because of your body size by friends, co-workers, or family:

_____

_____

Fat discrimination is very real in our society. The problem is especially frustrating because it seems virtually impossible to change the opinions of the thin world. How can they find out you are a worthwhile person if they don't give you a chance? Compare fat discrimination with racism.

8. Describe to what extent you feel your eating self-control is reduced by your negative moods (depression, PMS, worry, stress):

_____

_____

_____

_____

This can be a vicious cycle because your negative moods may be brought on or made worse by your negative emotional response to being overweight. Furthermore, because of fat discrimination, many overweight individuals feel under pressure to be happy and nice, in order to be less "offensive."

9. Write down your feelings about taking a very relaxed and very gradual approach to weight management:

_____

_____

_____

Try to relax, slow down, and have fun while learning to change your ways of thinking and behaving; achieve a managed weight which corresponds to better psychological as well as physical health.

2

IS OBESITY HEREDITARY?

About one quarter of adults in the United States are obese, making it a very common condition. Obesity means an excess of body fat. For most of us, our weight is a rough measure of how fat we are. If we weigh 20% or more than the height/weight tables say we should, the chances are that we are probably obese. Exceptions might include professional football players or some men who do strenuous physical labor for a living. These individuals may be heavier than the height/weight tables say they should be, but much of that heaviness is muscle. As a rule though, the tables are a fairly good guide for most of us.

Individuals who live in the Midwestern part of the United States are the heaviest.[1] The two states with the highest prevalence of obesity are Wisconsin (26%) and Indiana (26%). The two states with the thinnest people are New Mexico (15%) and Hawaii (16%). The South has the second highest prevalence of obesity, followed by the Northeast. The Western part of our country has the lowest amount of obesity. No one is exactly sure why obesity differs by state and by region. Perhaps the kinds or the amounts of food differ enough to account for the findings. Or perhaps levels of activity differ by area. Although all parts of this country have high levels of obesity, the Midwest does appear to be our *fat belt*.

Prevalence of obesity differs by race.[2] Black females in particular have very high levels, with over 60% in the 45 to 54 age range being overweight. This percentage remains relatively constant through age 74.

Poverty plays a role in obesity.[3] With men, there is a slightly higher prevalence of overweight at all ages among those above the poverty line. With women, the reverse is true. Women below the poverty line have a much higher prevalence of obesity at all ages, except ages 20-24. As men become richer, they tend to get heavier; as women get richer, they get thinner.

Obesity can be dangerous. The heavier a person is, the greater the chances of developing cardiovascular disease risk factors and some cancers. High blood pressure is three times more common in obese than normal weight individuals. High blood cholesterol is almost twice as prevalent in obese individuals than in those of normal weight (especially in younger people). Diabetes is three times higher in obese people. According to results from the Framingham Study, a large, long-term investigation, obesity is also an independent risk factor for coronary artery heart disease. Where the fat on the body is located may be particularly important. Too much fat around the waist (e.g., *beer bellies* or *pot bellies*) is more often related to diseases than fat in the lower body (e.g., thighs, hips, or buttocks). Upper-body fat appears to be the main killer.

Obese men have higher death rates from cancers of the colon, prostate, and rectum. Obese women have higher death rates from postmenopausal breast cancer and cancers of the gallbladder, uterus, and ovaries.

Obesity affects how long people live. The greater the obesity, the less the lifespan. Although some studies suggest that very thin weights are also related to higher death rates, closer analysis of the underweight individuals who died early suggest that many of the deaths were due to lung cancer, possibly associated with smoking. The increase in death rates in obese individuals is greater under the age of 50 years. Fat above the waist also is more predictive of death rates than fat below the waist.

It is clear that obesity can be dangerous to health and longevity. When weight is 20% or more above desirable, it appears to become a health problem.

THE ROLE OF GENETICS

Twins

Do individuals become heavy primarily because they have someone in their family tree who was heavy and who passed the obesity genes on to them? Or is development of the obese state primarily the result of environment, from eating too much and exercising too little? Dr. Claude Bouchard and his colleagues at Laval University in Quebec, Canada, recently tried to shed some light on the heredity question by recruiting 12 pairs of identical twins, 19 to 27 years old.[4] All of these monozygotic twins were males and each pair had been raised together and had been living together before the project. Thus each pair shared the same genes and the same environment.

The researchers locked up the twins in a college dormitory and watched them very closely during the 100 day study. The amount of exercise each subject was allowed to do was carefully supervised. The twins were first allowed to eat freely and their intake was measured. Once the researchers had determined the normal intake of each of the young men, they were fed their usual diet plus an additional 1,000 calories each day, six days a week, for the next 100 days. Each subject ate a total of 84,000 extra calories (that is, in addition to his usual diet).

All of the subjects gained weight during the study. The average weight gain was 18 pounds, but the range was enormous.

One subject gained only 9 1/2 pounds while another gained 29 pounds. What was most interesting was that the weight gains of each twin pair were much more similar than the gains between twin pairs. That is, the amount of variation within the twin pairs was only one third of the variation between the pairs. Other changes in fat followed the same pattern. The researchers concluded that the striking results were probably due to genetic factors which control our tendency to store energy as either fat or lean tissue and the determinants of the resting expenditure of energy.

In another study, using the Twin Registry maintained by the National Academy of Sciences-National Research Council, Dr. Albert Stunkard and his colleagues examined closely the heights and weights of 1,974 monozygotic and 2,097 dizygotic male twin pairs.[5] They found that the monozygotic twins were twice as similar as the dizygotic twins and that human fatness was under very strong genetic control. In an even more dramatic study of 93 identical twins who had been reared apart, Stunkard found that heredity accounted for about 70% of body fatness.[6]

Adoptees

The country of Denmark maintains a large adoption registry, listing every nonfamilial adoption granted between 1924 and 1947. The register contains information about both the adoptive parents and the biological parents. Using this register, scientists located and mailed a questionnaire to over 4,000 individuals who had been adopted during this period of time, asking for their heights and weights and other information. These adoptees were now adults with an average age of 42 years. Questionnaires were also mailed to both the adoptive and the biological parents, asking information about their heights and weights. The scientists then compared the weights of the adoptees with both their adoptive parents who raised them and their biological parents who had played no role in their upbringing. There was no relationship at all between the weights of the adoptees and their adoptive parents; there was a clear, strong relationship between the weights of the adoptees and their biologic parents across the whole range of body fatness, from the very thin to the very fat. The scientists concluded that genetic factors have an important influence on our fatness; family environment alone has no apparent effect at all.[7]

DOES METABOLISM PLAY A ROLE?

We do not know which genes cause obesity. However, we do know that a slow metabolism and a large number of fat cells can be inherited and probably play a major role in the development of obesity. Resting metabolic rate (RMR) means the energy needed to keep our heart beating, our blood pressure pumping, our breathing and our other vital functions working during the day. In sedentary people, that is, people who work at a desk all day and those who do not move around very much, resting metabolic rate accounts for about 70% of their daily energy expenditure. People with low energy expenditures do not burn many calories, those with high expenditures burn a large number. And wouldn't you know it, but our resting metabolic rate is inherited. Studies show that people with slow resting metabolic rates gain more weight than those with faster rates.[8,9] The more fat on a person, the slower the resting metabolic rate.

FAT CELL NUMBER

The normal-weight adult has about 30 billion fat cells, give or take 5 billion or so. We need some fat cells to store fat (triglyceride) for use under stress. As we grow older and get a little heavier, these fat cells tend to expand in size and weight. The term for this is *hypertrophy*. When we put on a moderate amount of weight, perhaps about 50 pounds or so, our number of fat cells also increases. In fact, in some individuals who gain a lot of weight, say over 150 pounds, the number of fat cells may increase to over 100 billion. The term for too many fat cells is *hyperplasia*. Severely obese people have too large fat cells (hypertrophy) and too many fat cells (hyperplasia). While it is possible to shrink fat cells by losing weight, it apparently is not possible to reduce the number of fat cells, which is why very fat people have a great deal of difficulty losing large amounts of weight. The size and the number of fat cells determine a person's lower weight range. These persons can only lower their weight by shrinking the size of their cells, not their number.

SET POINT

One useful way of putting all this information on genetics together is to use what is called a body *set-point*. Our bodies tend to defend a certain weight, that is, we can lower our weight by dieting for awhile, but with time the weight tends to return and we again weigh the same as before. This weight is known as our *set-point*. This set-point isn't really one number (like 187 pounds), but rather a range of pounds, over which we tend to fluctuate depending on our motivation, exercise, and eating patterns. The set point is really a combination of the size and number of our fat cells, our resting metabolic rate, and all of the other factors which contribute to our fatness. Set point can be a helpful shorthand term to describe all of these factors.

WEIGHT CYCLING

Repeated cycles of weight loss followed by weight regain may be harmful to our health.[10] Dr. Kelly Brownell and his colleagues examined the effects of weight fluctuation on adult male rats.[10] One group of rats was put on a high-fat diet until they became obese. They were then placed on a balanced eating plan and they returned to normal weight. This group was then allowed to eat the high-fat diet again and they, as before, became obese. One more time on the balanced diet and they returned to normal weight, followed by another regain on the high fat-diet. These animals therefore experienced two complete cycles of losing and gaining weight.

Results of the study were amazing. After becoming obese the first time, it took these rats 21 days to lose the weight. However, after they regained the weight, it took them 46 days to lose it again, even though the balanced diet was exactly the same each time.

How long did it take the rats to regain the weight? In the first cycle, they needed 45 days to return to their obese level after they came off their diet. In the second cycle, it took only 14 days to regain the same weight. Weight loss was twice as slow and weight regain was three times as fast during the second cycle.

Why? The rats seemed to be responding to dieting by becoming more efficient in their use of food. They gained more weight per ounce of food eaten during the second cycle and maintained their weight on fewer calories. This weight cycling appeared to increase the efficiency of the food eaten. With each cycle of loss and regain, the animals presumably were becoming more efficient, gaining on fewer calories, maintaining weight even with fewer calories coming in. This cycling behavior may even be contributing to the development of the obese state.

What are the implications for humans? Going on and off diets frequently, losing and regaining weight repeatedly, may make weight control much more difficult. Losing weight is serious business. Although Brownell's study is controversial, and much research is being conducted on the weight cycling question, our bodies probably are not built to lose and regain weight frequently. Losing weight permanently is not accomplished by going on and off diets.

IMPLICATIONS FOR THE OVERWEIGHT

What are the implications for overweight individuals with a family history of obesity, an excess number of fat cells, a high body set point, a low metabolic rate, or a history of weight cycling? What about the individual with all of these factors?

Results of studies are clear and unequivocal. There are strong and undeniable genetic influences on body fatness. Family environment alone does not seem to be a major factor in the development of obesity. What does this mean for people with genetic factors? Are all efforts doomed to failure for those genetically programmed to be obese?

Although genetic factors may explain much of the individual variation in fatness within our society, environmental influences also help account for some of the differences in fatness that occur among societies and social groups whose diets, activity levels, and attitudes about physical appearance differ. Prevalence of obesity in human populations is related to a number of factors, in addition to genetics, including social conditions and economic circumstances.

Individuals who have genetic factors predisposing them toward obesity will have a harder time trying to reach and maintain a lower weight. It is important to recognize that our weight is not simply due to how much we eat and exercise. Our knowledge of human obesity has progressed beyond these simple generalizations. Clearly, obesity has multiple causes and there are many different types. Regulation of weight is exceedingly complex. Our diets, exercise levels, attitudes, and feelings about ourselves all interact with genetic factors. All of us can look at ourselves, see what we can change, such as eating a healthy diet and getting regular exercise. We can learn to accept the limitations imposed on our weight management by those factors which we have little or no control. The purpose of this book is to help you achieve these goals.

THE BOTTOM LINE:

- Our genes affect our susceptibility toward obesity.

- Our diet and exercise level determine the expression of this susceptibility.

- We can all eat a healthful diet and exercise regularly, while learning to accept the genetic factors over which we have little or no control.

Awareness Exercises

1. Draw a family tree including your siblings, parents, aunts, uncles and grandparents. Who among these has a weight problem?

    _____

    _____

    _____

    If you find that many of your blood relatives are overweight, it may be due to either genetic factors or lifestyle similarities in eating and exercising.

2. Among those in your family who had a weight problem, did they get lots of regular exercise?

    _____

    _____

    _____

    You may find that relatives who exercise regularly tend to be thinner than those who do not.

3. Among those in your family with a weight problem, did they eat prudent, low-fat diets?

    _____

    _____

    You may find that relatives who avoid high-fat foods tend to be thinner than those who do not.

3

THE MIND VERSUS BODY

PROBLEM

The title of this chapter alludes to the fact that our bodies are designed to rebel against dieting, whether our minds want to succeed or not. Because of physiological (not psychological) factors, if you try to lose weight too fast, you just get stuck more tightly into a pattern of dieting, losing, and regaining. This up-down fluctuation in weight discussed in Chapter Two is known as the *yo-yo* effect. In order to explain the finger puzzle and yo-yo aspects of improper weight-management, we start with an old model of weight control and work up to a newer, more complex one. The old model looked like this:

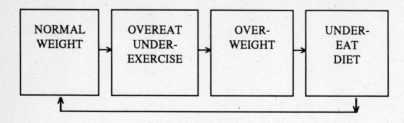

Old Model
Figure 3.1

The old model said, *Eat too much, get fat, diet, get thin.* But as many overweight persons know, it isn't that simple, and it certainly isn't that easy.

A more complex model is shown in Figure 3.2. It shows that a desire to be thin leads to dieting which leads to cravings and reduced self-control which lead to overeating which leads to a regain of lost weight and a need to repeat the cycle. Over time the problem gets worse, since during the cycle changes take place which make it easier for the body to store fat and harder to lose it.

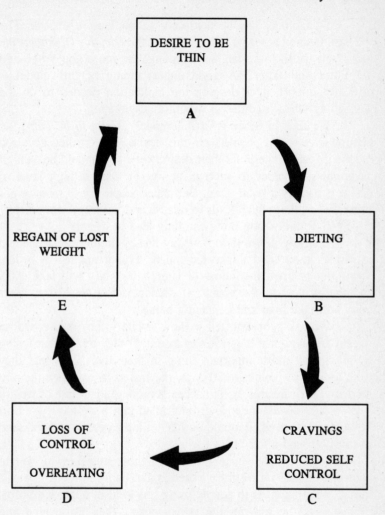

Dieter's Dilemma
Figure 3.2

This model has been around for at least a decade. Dr. William Bennett at Harvard has called it the *Dieter's Dilemma*: the more you try to lose weight by dieting, the more you yo-yo and get fatter and fatter.[1] A good understanding of this model is critically important to develop the motivation needed to do the right thing when it comes to weight management.

We start in Block A of this model, *Desire to be Thin*. We assume overweight people have this desire. But do they have too much? Most people think their desire to be thin should be as high as possible in order to succeed at weight loss. A high level of desire is usually a good thing. But many people try to lose weight using this model, which leads to relapse and failure. A very strong desire to do the wrong thing can only lead to trouble.

A strong desire to lose weight fast by dieting causes people to restrict their food intake too much. Trying not to eat is like trying not to breathe. Sooner or later, your body will take over, and you will gasp for breath. If dieting is too restrictive, your body will take over and demand a binge.

We ask people to tell us how strongly they desire to lose weight and how fast they want to lose it. If they tell us that losing weight is the most important thing in their lives, and that they want to lose 30 pounds in 30 days, our task is to convince them to moderate their desires, and to accept a more gradual rate of weight loss. If we allowed them to go unbridled into a weight-loss effort at too great a speed, it would be like telling a person in quicksand to move around a lot.

Most people make the two biggest mistakes in weight control: reliance on restrictive dieting and being in too much of a hurry. What happens to people using this kind of approach? Most of them end up playing the yo-yo game. They go around and around the cycle shown in Figure 3.2. Their weight cycles down and up again. For some, it might take several months to diet, relapse, and regain. For others, it might take what seems like a few days. What is the result of this endless game? People who play it end up feeling like failures, which reduces their self-esteem. Overweight people do not need further damage to their self-esteem. And, as we discuss in Chapter Four, reduced self-esteem goes hand in hand with negative emotions and reduced self-control.

In addition to psychological damage, playing this game also may lead to increased risk for diseases, thus adding injury to insult. Recent research has suggested that weight cycling may redistribute excess fat from the thighs to the middle.[2] This is thought to increase the risk for diabetes and heart disease. Another study found that people whose weight fluctuated over a period of years were more likely to suffer cardiovascular disease years later.[3] Apparently, weight cycling is not good for mind or body.

We continue through this new model step by step. Go to Block B, *Dieting*. Somewhere in the distant past humans got the idea that obesity was curable by eating less. It is true that a period of reduced eating will result in a period of reduced weight, but relapse makes the weight loss short-lived. A desire to be thin leads to restrictive dieting. A *restrictive* diet is one in which eating is consciously limited to less than is desired. Generally, if a person gets hungry on such a diet, and doesn't eat when hungry, it is restrictive.

Some restrictive diets involve eating grapefruit and celery. On others, eating is restricted to almost nothing on odd days, and eating is unlimited on even days. Other diets allow eating only tiny portions throughout the day. Most overweight people have suffered through three or more dieting efforts. Some have paid large sums of money to go to a very-low-calorie diet program, which requires medical supervision. Some have gone to a behavior modification program in which eating is controlled by changing the factors which affect eating behavior. The success rate of programs which restrict eating is less than 10 percent. By success we mean losing a meaningful amount of weight and keeping it off.

Why doesn't the weight stay off? The obvious reason for weight regain is a return to old eating and exercise habits. This takes us to Block C, *Cravings and Reduced Self-Control*. For those on a very restrictive diet, the body may rebel. Like persons who attempt breath holding, they may relapse quickly to out-of-control eating. It is now thought that restrictive dieting is one of the main causes of binge eating problems.[4] Others who diet may return to their former weights more gradually as their eating and exercise habits slowly return to former patterns. In any case, self-control seems to break down.

Researchers in Sweden found that dieters experiencing negative emotions or stress lost control of eating.[5] The dieters' thought processes about eating became irrational. Others have found that an overly restrictive diet can lead to depression.[6] Depression goes hand-in-hand with reduced self-control.

Studies of eating control relapse have shown that relapse is most likely when a dieter is alone and feeling down, or when feeling good at a party or restaurant.[7] Most relapses occur during late afternoon or evening. This may be due to the tendency of dieters to skip breakfast or to eat too little during the day. One study found that when breakfast was skipped, the chances of overeating at lunch were increased by 50 percent.[8] The sad news is that this same study found that overeating at a meal increased the probability of overeating at the next meal! Dieters can't win: Skip a meal and then overeat, or overeat and then overeat. It is easy to understand why overeating might occur after skipping a meal. Overeating after overeating occurs because many dieters feel that once they have *blown it* for a day, there is no use trying to restrict eating. Dieters usually tell themselves that they will start again on their diets tomorrow.

How can a person cope with such a conflict between desire to lose weight and uncontrolled eating? We tell our patients that one part of the brain controls logical thought. This part is saying, *I need to lose weight, and I must control my eating*. Another part of the brain controls eating. This eating control part is only slightly influenced by the thinking part of the brain. When it senses that the body is not getting enough food, it says, *I don't care what you're thinking, this body is going to eat!*

We think that this explanation is about as scientifically valid as any other theory which tries to explain irrational eating behavior. Scientists have yet to produce a good theory that explains the *Mind-Body Problem*. This is the problem of determining how thinking and consciousness relate to physiological activities and the subconscious. In the remaining chapters of this book we provide a plan which can work without requiring a good understanding of the Mind-Body Problem.

Let's move on to Block D of the Model, *Loss of Control and Overeating*. When a human is very hungry, a craving for high-fat foods arises. Such cravings may bring to mind french fries with gravy, chips, ice cream, enchiladas. The sad news is that restrictive dieting seems to increase cravings for calorie-dense foods. This would be adaptive if we lived in the wilderness where food was very scarce. In that situation, we would be thankful to be automatically programmed by nature to eat an abundance of high-fat food, since we might not eat so well again for a long time. However, with high-fat foods now available everywhere, these cravings work against us.

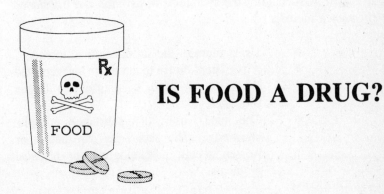

IS FOOD A DRUG?

As humans we are programmed to enjoy eating. The act of eating releases morphine-like chemicals to the brain, which explains why eating is a pleasurable experience. Sex and exercise do the same thing. For many overweight persons, especially those who have a history of repeatedly trying to lose weight through restrictive dieting, the eating of food results in consequences that go far beyond the normal satisfaction derived from eating. Such persons may discover that eating can temporarily relieve them from feelings of depression, anxiety, or anger. This is especially dangerous if one of the reasons for being depressed, anxious and angry is the fact that they are overweight.

If overweight persons discover that a behavior or substance makes them feel better, they can become psychologically dependent upon that behavior or substance. For example, if a person has problems in her life that are depressing, and she feels better after smoking marijuana, the relief from psychological suffering can be so reinforcing that she may make smoking marijuana a regular habit. She can become dependent upon the drug to help her deal with negative emotions. The anxiety and fear of facing life without marijuana is so threatening that it becomes very difficult to stop using it, even though it may not be physically addicting.

It can happen with eating, too. According to the American Psychiatric Association,[9] the symptoms of *psychoactive substance dependence* include:

- Using more of the substance than intended.
- A persistent desire to cut down and repeated efforts to cut down or control use of the substance.
- Continued use of substance despite knowledge that such use can cause or worsen social, psychological, or physical problems.

- Negative emotions associated with not using substance (withdrawal).
- Substance often taken to relieve or avoid withdrawal symptoms.

When the psychiatrists developed this list of symptoms, they had in mind substances like alcohol, cocaine, or marijuana, which can alter consciousness and change mood. We feel that many overweight persons suffer from food dependence. Substitute the word *food* for *substance* in the above list of symptoms. The result is:

- Unintended overeating.
- Desire to lose weight and repeated dieting.
- Inability to control eating.
- Feeling bad when on a restrictive diet.
- Overeating when feeling sad, mad, or scared.

Among overweight persons who seek treatment, about 50 percent report having at least weekly episodes of uncontrolled, excessive eating. Another 30 percent have these periods of out-of-control eating less frequently.[10] If persons overeat two or more times each week, and feel out of control during these binges, they may have *nonpurging bulimia*. Persons with this disorder have more difficulty controlling weight, since they are more out of control. However, as the label implies, they do not purge (vomit, or abuse laxatives or diuretics).

For some overweight people, food may be used as a *drug*. Stress, frustration, rejection, and other negative emotions have been found to precede uncontrolled binges, and the binge seems to bring temporary relief from these negative feelings.[11] Excessively restrictive dieting can add to the negative feelings, so that a binge can be triggered by excessive hunger as well as the need to soothe oneself with the *drug* of food.

This does not mean that an individual has an addiction to food. For example, there is no evidence for addiction to any particular food such as sugar or white flour, even though some people swear they have such addictions.[12] An addiction implies a disease state in which the body is susceptible to a particular substance. We define food dependence as a state of relying on food to feel better. This can be treated by helping individuals change their thoughts and feelings about being overweight, and altering eating and exercise patterns.

Binge eating usually involves foods high in both carbohydrates and fat. Research has shown that in many cases obesity may be related to a high fat-to-carbohydrate ratio in the diet rather than to overeating.[13] If a person eats few carbohydrates (beans, pastas, grains, starches) and too many high-fat foods, the appetite control mechanisms may cause consumption of too many calories. If the consumption of carbohydrates is high (according to the plan described in Chapter Eight), you may be able to lose weight by reducing the fat content of your diet.[14] A study by Dr. David Levitsky and his colleagues at Cornell University showed that women could lose weight by eating a diet which had 22 percent of calories from fat without a need to eat less than they desired.[15] Thus the key to avoiding yo-yo dieting may be to reduce fat in the diet without feeling deprived.

Overeating by itself can lead to overweight, but overeating high-fat foods is a double whammy. First, fat is high calories. Second, fat calories seem to contribute to obesity more than do calories from carbohydrates or protein.

The problem is that negative emotions about being overweight trigger dieting, which can trigger negative emotions, which trigger binges, which trigger negative emotions about binging, leading to a vicious cycle. In the next few chapters we show how to break free of this cycle.

Judy

Judy is a 40-year-old housewife, married to an engineer. They have three children. Judy has had a weight problem since she was 13. Here is some of what she wrote during treatment:

About age thirteen I began to put on more than curves. I guess I became less active and more 'lady-like' at the same time. I began to feel pudgy, especially with water weight around my periods. I did what everyone else did, I dieted. My dieting was mainly an effort to eat less. I skipped meals, and avoided bread, potatoes, and desserts. I know now this wasn't very sound nutritionally, but in my family we grew up on a high-fat diet of fried foods, whole dairy products, and 'dessert' seemed like one of the major food groups, since we had dessert with almost every meal.

Nobody in my family exercised as far as I can remember. Neither of my parents was terribly fat, just a little thick in the middle. My two sisters never had a problem with weight. They are older than I am, and still don't have a problem even after having kids. It is a mystery to me. I used to think there was something wrong with me, being the only fat kid in the family.

I do remember that my sisters weren't very interested in cooking; they were really tomboys until their late teens. Mom shared most of her cooking knowledge with me. We were a great cooking team. Of course, she knew nothing of nutrition and that's why our meals were so high in fat. I think that my relationship with food started then, just before I started dieting. I realize now that I was already developing a love-hate relationship with food. I was learning how to cook and serve food, to make it more attractive, while at the same time I was learning how to avoid food.

I went on and off countless diets like lots of people. My weight problem gradually got worse over the years. I sure wish I could live my teen-age years again as a thin person! By adulthood, I was about 50 pounds over what I wanted to be. I managed to lose about 30 pounds for a while, and got married. But having three kids took its toll. I quickly got back to my highest weight and stayed there for years.

Ever since I can remember, at least from my teen years, I have thought about my weight problem every day. I often have fantasies about what it would be like to be thin. I have had some dreams about being thin. The funny thing is, in my dreams there is a 'Prince Charming,' but it is all very scary, I guess because I'm not sure I would know how to handle the attention. My husband loves me but I always feel that it could be a lot better romantically and sexually if I could just be thin. I try to accept that I may never be thin, but fantasies and daydreams can be fun. I mean, I am too old now to expect a torrid romance. I try to explain this to my daughters but I don't want them to diet like I did.

What I am learning in this program is that I will lose the battle if I am at war with myself. If I am in a hurry to lose weight, and my goal weight is too low, I will just be in a tug of war with myself. My desire to control my eating will fight with my increasing cravings to eat the wrong foods. When I eat, I will enjoy the foods but feel shame and guilt for eating them. You can't win if the war is inside yourself. I will try to slow down and to accept a weight goal of 160, but it won't be easy. I hope what you say about gradual change of attitudes and group support works with me! I have been depressed about my appearance for years. I don't need another failure. Help!

Progress: Judy has been trying to exercise regularly, and to eat alternative, lower-fat foods. Her husband has agreed to let her have at least three evenings a week for exercise and getting away from the kids. She appears to be enjoying the camaraderie of the support group. At this time, the group is trying to motivate

Judy to slow down her weight loss to less than one pound per week. She had wanted to lose two pounds per week, since that was the goal in her last weight-loss attempt at a clinic.

THE BOTTOM LINE:

- Never diet again; reduce fat in your eating instead.

- Take your weight management plan slowly.

- You may have developed a food dependence.

- Don't blame yourself for being out of control after dieting. Your body was designed to eat after dieting just as it was designed to gasp for air after restricted breathing.

Awareness Exercises

1.   Have you found dieting to be less enjoyable and more difficult to do over the years? Describe your experiences.

_____

_____

_____

After many diets, your body may change in ways that make sticking to a diet and keeping weight off more difficult. Certainly after many failures, your self-confidence can be destroyed.

2.   Multiply the number of pounds you want to lose by 1.2. The answer equals the number of weeks required to lose this weight gradually. Pounds to lose _____ X 1.2 = _____ weeks. Describe your feelings about having to wait this long to lose this much weight.

_____

_____

_____

_____

There is no quick cure for weight management. Slow to gain, slow to lose. The faster you lose, the easier it is to relapse and regain. Most successful weight managers have taken the slow way.

3.　Describe how your self-esteem has been hurt by your failure to manage your weight.

_____

_____

_____

_____

Most people's self-esteem is tied in part to their feelings about their appearance, since our culture is obsessed with "looking good." If you think it's your fault that you can't stay thin, then you may feel like a failure as well as feeling unattractive.

4.　The success rate of diet programs is less than 10 percent. Do you think you will try another one knowing how low your chances are of achieving satisfactory results?

_____

_____

_____

Sometimes in desperation people will grab at any opportunity even if the chances for success are slim. But if you have tried many times without success, it may be time to consider another way.

5.   Binging may be caused by dieting. Do you think that you
      may sometimes overeat because of not eating enough?
      Describe your experiences.

      _____

      _____

      _____

      _____

      *Do you binge because you are overly hungry? Are you
      overly hungry because you haven't been eating enough?
      Have you been dieting to lose the weight you gained from
      your last binges? Do you want to stop this vicious cycle?*

6.   What are your relapse risks? Anger? Depression? PMS?
      Loneliness? Parties? Write down the conditions you feel
      are related to your loss of eating control.

      _____

      _____

      _____

      _____

      *Remember that you may never be free of the emotions
      related to anger, depression or PMS. However, there are
      strategies to reduce the tendency to lose control: avoid
      dieting, get peer support. It is far from hopeless.*

7.   Describe how much you are bothered by not being able to control your eating.

_____

_____

_____

_____

To a large extent, trying to "control" your eating is like trying to control your breathing. Don't blame yourself for the body's natural response to dieting.

8.   Does eating sometimes make you feel better when you are down or nervous? Is food a drug for you?

_____

_____

_____

Eating has a calming effect on animals. It can be especially calming after nervousness related to dieting. You are probably not a "food addict" any more than you would be an "air addict" by gasping for breath after shallow breathing. Thus, food may not be like a drug, but eating may have a drug-like effect.

4

LOOKISM AND THE OBESE SELF

Lookism: The belief that appearance is an indicator of a person's value; the construction of a standard of beauty/attractiveness; and oppression through stereotypes and generalizations of both those who do not fit that standard and those who do.[1]

...behold, all is vanity and a striving after wind.[2]

And remember friends, it's better to look good than to feel good.[3]

Who is a Lookist? If individuals are concerned about the way they look due to being overweight, then they are lookists. Many people, women in particular, have accepted society's standards of attractiveness and acceptable body size. They have failed to meet these standards, and they are upset about it.

Only one hundred years ago, plumpness was fashionable. *Fat-Ten-U* brand foods were *guaranteed to make the thin Plump and Comely*. The beauties depicted in the paintings of Peter Paul Rubens would today be diagnosed as obese and in desperate need of treatment. There are still cultures in which women must be quite fat before they are acceptable as brides. At the beginning of this century, thinness was associated with the lower classes who were thin due to poverty and/or a lifestyle which included much labor-intensive house or farm work. Others were thin from tuberculosis and other health problems.

Something happened between then and now. After World War I, the advent of mass production of fashionable women's apparel in standard sizes, together with mass media photography depicting *fashionable* celebrities, quickly spread the new standards of beauty throughout the land. In the Roaring Twenties, outward appearance became more important than inner character because sexual attractiveness had replaced spirituality as the most important attribute of a woman.[4]

The mass production of clothes and appearance-enhancing products made it possible for the masses to participate in fashion. Advertising emphasized that such products were absolutely necessary to achieve the proper look. The message was clear: unless you adhered to the standards of slenderness and fashion, you would not be loved or respected.

A recent issue of a popular women's magazine had advertisements for the following products:

- make-up
- perfume
- skin-firming concentrate
- prosthetic eyelashes
- bust firming gel
- cellulite control gel
- night repair lotion

- self-tanning moisturizers
- anti-aging cream
- hair shampoos/conditioners/rinses/colorings/highlighters
- stress cream
- fashions
- figure-modifying undergarments

The message underlying these ads is *You are not good enough without a lot of help*. There were also products advertised which undoubtedly are damaging to appearance: cigarettes and alcohol. On the other hand, some ads were for fitness equipment and exercise shoes. There was even a feature article on the dangers of narcissism. But on the whole, the advertising and articles of many women's magazines reflect a high and continuing demand for products designed to mask a person's true appearance. The products sell because many women find their natural appearance to be unacceptable.

All these products are supposed to make one sexier. Women are led to believe that if they are sexually attractive, they will be wanted, or at least their bodies will be wanted. Most American women believe that all parts of their body need to be smaller, except their breasts.[5] Most women believe that they are well above their ideal weight, and heavier than the weight that would make them most attractive to men. But most men think women would be most attractive to them at a size which is larger than women's imagined attractive weight.[6]

Many men are attracted to female breasts and buttocks. These body parts get their shape and size from fat. At the same time a woman is trying to be thin, she might want to leave these parts fat. But it is difficult to lose fat selectively. This problem has led to a booming business in plastic surgery. According to the American Society of Plastic and Reconstructive Surgeons, Inc., over 620,000 *aesthetic surgery procedures* are performed each year in the U.S.A. These involve modifications of the breast, cheek, chin, ears, eyelids, face, hips, abdomen, and buttocks.

No one seems to be satisfied with their own body. Many white people want to be darker, even though tanning is now known to be a cause of skin cancer. People with straight hair want to have curly hair. Some black people want to be lighter and have straight hair. Overweight people want to be thin. Thin women want bigger breasts. A poll showed that 96 percent of Americans wanted to change something about their bodies.[7]

Yet the relationship between appearance and happiness is far from clear. Getting the body one desires doesn't necessarily produce the expected results. There are disadvantages to being good-looking.[8] Beautiful women are often spoiled as children, and people react to their beauty instead of their personality. Some of the most beautiful women we have had as patients in psychotherapy had extreme difficulty with personal relationships and romance; they were confused and depressed. Some men who have relations with beautiful women feel more insecure because they think that other males are plotting to take their women away from them. This insecurity can drive them to extreme possessiveness, making for a very sick relationship.

Unattractive or overweight people may feel ashamed of their appearance; beautiful people may feel self-conscious. Ordinary-looking persons wish they were more attractive. It might be psychologically more healthful if everyone in our society were blind.

Coping With Overweight In a Lookist Society

One problem an overweight person may have is: *How do I cope successfully with my weight problem?* The word *successfully* implies a coping method which will bring happiness. Many people feel the way to cope with overweight is to become thin. But they haven't been able to achieve thinness. As discussed in Chapter

Two, genetic inheritance, childhood family practices and a history of dieting may have led to an excessive number of fat cells in the body so that thinness is not a realistic option any more.

Coping Method One: Continue to Be Upset about Being Overweight and Try to Lose More Fat

This coping method is responsible for the cycle of dieting/overexercising, binging and regain discussed in Chapter Three. In Figure 3.2, we showed how a desire to be thin led to dieting which led to loss of control. There is another dimension to this cycle which is depicted in Figure 4.1. Many overweight people believe that their weight problem affects their self-worth and self-esteem, and inhibits others from giving them the love they desire. Because they have fallen for the lookist cult of appearance, they believe that they must lose weight to be loved. This places a tremendous amount of pressure on them to lose weight.

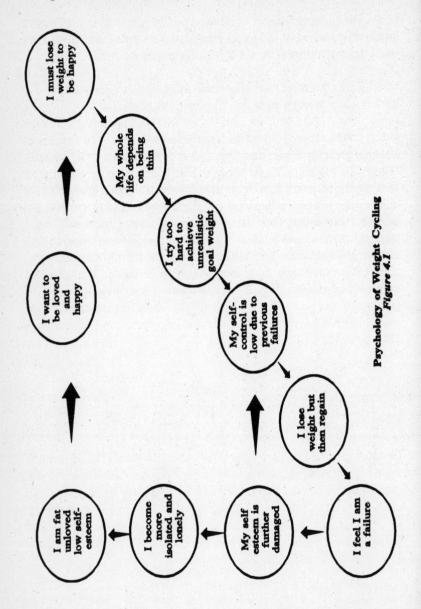

Psychology of Weight Cycling
Figure 4.1

Many thin people think that overweight people don't have enough willpower to lose weight. On the contrary, we think that one of the problems of overweight persons is that they seem to have too much willpower. They are able to force their bodies into very restrictive diets and/or very strenuous exercise regimens because of their obsession with weight loss.

But eventually the body rebels against this willpower. Lapse and relapse occur. They begin their efforts with high enthusiasm. As they feel themselves slipping, their enthusiasm turns to self-doubt. They have failed to achieve lasting weight loss before; they begin to feel that they have faltered again. These thoughts of failure, fed by their underlying low self-esteem as an obese person, eat away at self-confidence. As self-confidence diminishes, self-control, or *willpower*, fades. As self-control fades, physiology takes over. Relapse and regain are now assured.

Thus overweight individuals feel like failures. This further reduces self-esteem, making self-control even more difficult to achieve in the next attempt. They end up more discouraged, more isolated and unloved. After a period of self-hatred and depression, they are ready to begin the cycle again.

Coping Method Two: Fighting Society

There is a growing movement, led mostly by women, to combat the prejudices against the overweight. As Susie Orbach has pointed out, discrimination against fat people is a feminist issue.[9] Females are controlled by a male-dominated society in which women are brought up to believe that appearance is of the utmost importance. Females are made to feel inadequate through the use of unrealistically thin and beautiful models. Feelings of inadequacy in females put males at an advantage in social and sexual interactions. Thinner women also play this game to get advantage over their heavier sisters.

We agree that body size discrimination is unfair and unjust. But before anyone becomes involved in a feminist-political movement, she should be aware of the costs involved. One's motivation to use this coping method may be anger. Anger is usually not a good motivator. Sustained anger may lead to stress disorders. The many battles she may lose on the way to winning the war may lead to depression. Anyone taking this path should be sure to enlist plenty of social support.

We refer female readers to the feminist resources listed in Appendix B. We only advise that love can be more influential than anger, and less harmful. This advice applies to men as well as women.

Coping Method Three: Make Being Overweight Acceptable

Many overweight people are going to remain heavy for the rest of their lives. Regardless of exercise and diet changes, they reach a limit of fat loss which cannot be crossed without unhealthful starvation. Achieving happiness without ever being thin requires learning to accept extra fat. Many overweight persons hate their bodies. They get angry at their thighs. Hating parts of one's body is not conducive to psychological health. In order to accept an overweight body, therapists now advise the obese person to make peace with these body parts. The hate relationship is recognized. Experiential exercises are done to help in bodily self-acceptance. For example, body parts are viewed in a mirror while the owner thinks about them in a kinder way. *These are the thighs which support me*, rather than *Why can't my thighs lose fat when I diet?* Numerous books on this topic have been published in the last ten years, some of which are listed in Appendix B.

This method follows the prayer: *Help me to accept the things I cannot change.* In order to accept themselves as heavy forever, overweight persons must first go through a grieving process to say good-bye to the thin self they will never attain.

Otherwise, they will be continually reverting back to their old dieting ways with yo-yo weight fluctuations and ultimate failure to make any significant changes. Dr. Donna Ciliska's approach[10] includes coping with the sense of loss that comes with the realization that one will most likely never be thin.

Many find it helpful to join with other like-minded overweight persons to learn to accept their bodies as they are. This reduces the pressure to diet, which only leads to frustration and despair. The National Association for the Advancement of Fat Acceptance (NAAFA) is working to help those struggling with self-acceptance as fat persons. NAAFA also is active in fighting against fat discrimination. Their address is listed in Appendix B.

Coping Method Four: Making Appearance Irrelevant

This is the most difficult coping method, but it is the one most likely to bring fulfillment and happiness. It is difficult because it calls for an end to judging people on the basis of appearance. This is almost impossible in a lookist culture. This must be done even though overweight people have been conditioned over their entire lives to be aware of what other people look like, and to be painfully self-conscious of their own appearance.

We believe that for overweight persons to achieve this goal they need a philosophy of life which gives them a sense of direction. They need a philosophy which forms a solid foundation for their belief that the value of persons lies in their character, not in their appearance. The major religions provide a basis for such a philosophy. Religions such as Judaism, Christianity, and Buddhism emphasize that we should all love one another as we love ourselves. Compassion is the guiding principle. Our philosophy of life should be that all our behavior is directed toward:

- The nurturing and development of ourselves, and
- The nurturing and development of others.

These goals should be balanced. Our resources should be divided between self and others so that we get enough to survive and be happy, and then we give our extra resources and energy for others.

There is no room for lookism in a life directed by a religion or philosophy based on such goals. Lookism is a system for discrimination, for withholding of nurturing, and for the thwarting of personal development. Lookism ostracizes and rejects; love invites and accepts.

If *religion* is a negative word, consider the psychological research on happiness. Researchers have studied happy people, and have found that they share some common attitudes and behaviors. These researchers have also trained others to have these attitudes and behaviors. The trainees report being happier after their training. Many people believe you can't achieve happiness by trying to be happy, but you can if you try the correct method.

Some of the common attitudes and behaviors shared by happy people are:

- Be active and busy. Avoid TV and other passive entertainments. Spend free time nurturing yourself and others.

- Spend more time socializing. Sharing with others is very important.

- Be organized. Keep a list of goals. Plan your time on a calendar.

- Be productive at meaningful work. Try to have a job that is valuable to you, your company, and to society.

- Be realistic in your goals. Lower your expectations. You won't be able to get everything you want out of life, such as a thin body.

- Do what you can to have close relationships. This is one of the most important factors for happiness.

- Focus on the positive. View life as a series of opportunities and growth experiences, even though some may involve pain. Avoid worrying, anger, depression.

It is important to notice that none of the characteristics of happiness depend upon appearance or degree of overweight. Society may have conditioned overweight individuals to believe that happiness was something given only to the thin. We feel that the overweight can be happier if they follow the principles of happiness or of their religion and use the methods for eating and exercise control described in this book. Resources on happiness are listed in Appendix B.

In Chapter One we outlined this approach. In Chapter Two we discussed the results of scientific research on the causes of obesity. In Chapter Three we examined the vicious cycles which keep the obese trapped in a no-win situation. This chapter has explained how lookism motivates the thin to reject the overweight and how it causes the overweight to reject themselves. Lookist attitudes are the psychological driving force behind diet-relapse cycles.

The Obese Self

An *obese self* is one which adheres to the values of a lookist society. As a consequence, an obese self feels rejected and experiences self-hatred.

What is the answer? We recommend striving to achieve a *healthy self*. The characteristics of the *obese self* and the *healthy self* are contrasted in Table 4.1.

TABLE 4.1
THE OBESE SELF VS. THE HEALTHY SELF

THE OBESE SELF	THE HEALTHY SELF
Lookist attitudes	Nurturant attitudes
Social isolation	Social immersion
Self-rejection	Self-acceptance
Dieting/relapse cycles	Eats prudently
No exercise or overdoes and relapses	Moderate exercise
Focuses on mistakes; Feels like failure	Mistakes seen as learning experiences
Uses obesity as excuse for failures in life	Obesity not allowed to interfere with life
Focuses on past	Focuses on present
Negative emotions reduce self-control	Positive attitude helps self-control
Victim	Victor
Focuses on appearance	Focuses on health
Wants to improve appearance to get nurturance	Wants health to be active in nurturant relationships

In order to escape from the obese self, overweight individuals must direct their energies into developing and maintaining mutually nurturing relationships. They must immerse themselves in social activities rather than in isolation. They must learn to accept themselves regardless of their body size. Persons who feel they are failures because of an apparent inability to control their weight need to focus on feelings of success in relationship building. They need to focus on what they can do now to build these relationships rather than letting their feelings of depression from past failures and rejection overwhelm them. They must learn that happiness comes from good relationships and that happiness can engender greater self-control. They must stop feeling like victims, and start acting like victors.

The key to all of this is to immerse oneself into a social support system where one can learn new ways of relating, and new ways of thinking about oneself. This is the subject of Chapter Five.

Cynthia

Cynthia is a 35-year-old accountant. She weighed 185 pounds, and is 5'6" tall. She came to treatment after failure at several diet-based programs and considerable fluctuation in weight. She was binge eating about two times per week, usually on the weekends. She was mildly depressed, and complained about never having any close relationships because of being overweight. She wrote the following as part of her therapy:

I have been pretty heavy ever since I can remember. I can remember the kids teasing me in first grade. I don't have any painful emotional memories until I was 10 years old, in fourth grade, when I was excluded from a group of female friends because I was too fat. I should also mention that my brother and two sisters are normal weight. I am beginning to realize that my mother paid more attention to them, probably because of my weight. Everyone in my family was normal or thin. My father was very successful and mom and dad put a lot of effort into presenting themselves in the best way. We belonged to the country club set, I guess you could say.

I recall my mother fussing a lot about my appearance, not criticizing my weight directly, but making sure I dressed right and used makeup correctly. As a young teenager I saw my friends use what I thought was a lot of makeup and dress provocatively. I felt strange putting on makeup and trying to look good, since I felt so basically unattractive due to being heavy. No one said I had a pretty face, either. Mother kept telling me 'A girl has to make the best of what she has.' (As I am writing this, I feel some anger about dear old mom!) I suppose mom was realistic about my chances for dating, since she never pushed it or said anything about my not dating. My brother and sisters were somewhat active in dating. It was just an unsaid assumption that I was not going to be dating since I was too fat. I even considered a way to meet a boy at school who was also overweight, but he was such a geek. I also thought it would be ridiculous for us to be seen together.

Mom subscribed to all the fashion magazines. I remember reading them in my room and fantasizing how it would be if I were thin. I used to admire the models. But I always suspected that they were thin because they were starving themselves or were taking pills. On the other hand, I felt I was fat because I was lazy and I couldn't stick to a diet. I have seen the magazines they have today for fat women, with fat models, even fatter than me. I agree with what they are saying, but I guess I was so well trained by my mother that I still have a hard time accepting that being overweight is anything but unattractive.

I feel that I am an intelligent woman and very capable of loving someone dearly but who am I kidding. I can't get a date. I dress in dark unrevealing clothing. I seldom go out. When I do, I sit in the corner, out of any bright lights. I can't help feeling that the thin people look at me like I was wearing a clown suit. I know this is my imagination but it still hurts.

Progress: Cynthia has developed some friends in the support group. She has been able to identify with the characteristics of the *obese self* listed in Table 4.1. Being in the group is helping her to focus on relationships and worry less about appearance. She was raised in the Christian church and is being urged to look at her attitudes about her appearance from a spiritual standpoint. She is learning to enjoy social outings with her group members because they can talk about how it feels to be self-conscious about being overweight while they are in a public setting.

THE BOTTOM LINE:

• Individuals may look better and have better control of their weight if they put more energy into health and relationships.

• The first step in having energy for nurturant relationships is to accept yourself as you are.

Awareness Exercises

1. Describe how you felt about your appearance as a child and as a teenager. Write down any memories of social rejection.

    _____

    _____

    _____

    Most individuals who have been overweight since childhood have a long list of painful memories. Being cut off from friendship and love because of appearance rather than because of character is doubly painful because it seems so unjust.

2. Describe your feelings about your appearance as an adult.

    _____

    _____

    _____

    When you look at your feelings about your appearance, are you comparing yourself to thinner people? Can you look at your own features and see an interesting and worthwhile human being who can stand alone without invidious comparisons?

3.   List here all the negative thoughts you have had about your appearance. Describe the problems you feel you have with your thighs, hips, stomach, breasts, arms, face, hair.

_____

_____

_____

_____

Ask yourself how many people fit all the standards of beauty mandated by our culture. Not very many. It is obvious that many people would be happier if these standards were relaxed, if not ignored.

4.   List here all the products you can find in your home which you use to enhance your appearance.

_____

_____

_____

_____

Do the advertisements for these products carry the message that you aren't good enough in some way without using the product? You bought the product. Do you buy the message?

5. How much time do you spend each day working on your appearance?

_____

The average American female spends 45 minutes getting ready for each day.

6. Describe what improvements you would like to have in your appearance if a fairy godmother could magically make any changes.

_____

_____

_____

7. What movie stars would you most like to resemble?

_____

_____

_____

8.   Describe your feelings about the high probability that you may never look much better than you do now.

_____

_____

_____

_____

Look at your answers to numbers 6,7, and 8. Do you think fantasies about impossible goals are helpful or do you think it is better to face the truth and learn to accept it?

9.   Reflecting back over your life, what do you feel has brought you greater happiness: Looking good or good relationships? Discuss this.

_____

_____

_____

_____

_____

You will never have peace without love. You may never have love if concern for appearance comes first.

5

SOCIAL SUPPORT

No person is an island.[1]

Two are better than one, because they have a good reward for their toil. For if they fall, one will lift up the other; but woe to those who are alone when they fall and have not another to lift them up.[2]

We live in a culture which idealizes thinness and ostracizes on the basis of fatness. This is a very sad situation for those who seem unable to become thin. The prejudice against the overweight may lead to social isolation starting in childhood. This may affect the development of social skills. An obese person may end up isolated, depressed, and without the self-esteem and social skills needed to cultivate friendships.

This is being borne out in research. Depression is twice as prevalent in women as in men. One of the explanations for this is that women are made to feel inadequate for failing to achieve the cultural ideal of thinness.[3] Depression and social isolation go hand-in-hand. A study in Sweden found that overweight adults were significantly less likely to socialize with friends, go to the movies, eat in a restaurant, or go on trips.[4] In another study in Vermont, obese and non-obese women conversed by telephone. Judges, who did not know the weight status of the women, listened to audio tape recordings of the conversations. They rated the obese women as less likeable, less physically attractive, and with inferior social skills.[5] The judges probably rated the obese this way because the obese subtly communicated their lower self-esteem in their manner of talking.

In Chapter Four we pointed out that one important part of the cycle of weight loss attempts and relapse was that low self-esteem and negative emotions seemed to damage self-control. Further, low self-esteem leads to social isolation; social isolation can lead to depression; and depression damages self-esteem. Each failed attempt to control weight makes these factors worse.

The answer to this dilemma requires reaching out for social support. Research clearly shows that people with social support are better able to maintain weight loss than those without it.[6,7] Therefore, in this chapter we will emphasize the critical need for social support.

Care must be exercised when selecting social support persons. You can't get social support from just anybody. If you were to pick someone out of a crowd, he or she might support the prejudices against obesity. The support you would get from such a person might be *Eat less. Show a little more willpower.* This advice would only add to the problem.

But suppose you were able to find individuals who had problems similar to yours. Individuals who had found ways of coping with overweight which led to greater happiness and health. These are the type of mentors needed. Individuals who know what they are talking about because they have lived it. Individuals who know the psychological pain you may now be experiencing.

How Social Support Works

In Chapter One, we alluded to social support as a way of using someone else's rational thinking when your ability to think clearly was reduced by food cravings or negative emotions. We also talked about the forest ranger who was more likely to do the socially correct behavior if company was coming. Social support has many other features which can be helpful in getting out of the low self-esteem/depression/low social-skills pattern that many overweight people find themselves in after years of unsuccessful weight management efforts. Social support has been studied in small groups of people helping each other to control eating and other addictions.[8] There are numerous ways this kind of support can help.

Of course, not everything that works for one person is guaranteed to work for another person; people are different. But you will find what works for you, and support people can help you find your own unique ways of acting and thinking based on their own experience.

The most obvious way others can help is to give *advice* on what to do. You can learn from others who have *been there* and who have successfully coped with their problems. For example, they can teach what you need to do to resist urges to diet. This helps you have hope; if they can do it, so can you. They can also practice these methods with you. This can give a feeling of self confidence to know that what you are doing has worked for others. Compare this with trying to do everything on your own; feelings of self-doubt are bound to come up: *Am I doing the right thing? I am probably doing this the wrong way.* These are the kinds of thought patterns which arise if you have a history of failure in weight management efforts.

When you falter, support people are there to comfort and encourage you to keep on going. When you succeed, they will be there to give praise. This will help to prevent damage to self-esteem from failures, and will boost self-esteem with every success. This is needed to help end the tendency to put yourself down, which only leads to reduced self-esteem and less self-control.

Another important feature of support is that others who have won the battle can *share the emotions and experiences* they have had. This lets you know that you are not alone in the pain and struggles you may be having. This lets you know that you are *normal*. If you felt that you were the only person with such emotions, you might tend to suspect that you were different; this would tend to damage self-esteem even further.

When making changes in lifestyle, you must face the truth. This can be very painful. Left on your own, you might avoid dealing with issues which affect eating and exercise control. For example, if you were abused as a child, this may have a damaging effect on your self-esteem as an adult; this would make eating control more difficult. The best kind of support persons will put pressure on you to reveal things about yourself you might want to keep hidden. Support persons can help get the pain of your childhood out into the open so that you can vent your anger, forgive the abuser, and get on with life.

Just talking about eating and exercise problems with support persons helps *organize your thoughts* about your situation. Explaining yourself to others helps to get a perspective. If you do not communicate to others, all the emotions and thoughts you have tend to be jumbled together, adding to confusion and anxiety. Writing a diary which you share with support persons is an excellent idea.

If you have low self-esteem, it may be because you have ideas and feelings which are unrealistically negative. You may have been trying to improve self-esteem by striving in vain to succeed at weight control. You may have been thinking, *When I get control of my eating, then I will be a better person.* But continued failure in this effort only reduces self-esteem. When you get to know support persons, they will give *honest feedback* about you which will be more realistic. This feedback can help you reformulate self-attitudes and help to boost self-esteem. Support persons can assure you that you can have success, to boost self-confidence.

When you tell your eating and exercise goals to support persons, you put yourself under constructive social pressure to meet your goals. This is like a forest ranger asking people to visit frequently so that he will be motivated to bathe regularly. You will want to be able to report that you did what you said you would do. This is very different from the social pressure from our culture, which demands thinness through dieting. Your support persons will help you follow a non-diet plan which is gradual and minimizes relapse. They will help you through crises rather than reject you for failures.

When you stray from the plan by eating too little or too much a support group can help carefully analyze what happened, and help work out an alternative strategy to avoid the causes of the lapse. This kind of support helps you to continue in your efforts.

The most important help a support person can give is to *lend emotional support and a clear-thinking brain* when you are having a temptation crisis. A temptation crisis is any situation in which you feel that you may stray from the plan, either by returning to dieting or by binging. As we discussed in Chapter Three, weight management can be viewed as a battle between the body and the mind. Even when following the gradual plan we recommend in Chapter Eight, you may be tempted to return to old patterns. Using a friend to talk you through a crisis may be the most critical method of weight management you can ever learn. If you try to cope with crises all by yourself, you may fail, putting yourself into the downward spiral of failure, reduced self-esteem, and further loss of control. Reaching out to others increases chances of success. It also provides the opportunity to make your friends happier knowing they have helped someone.

A group can be very effective in keeping you on the right track by setting up certain rules and procedures. One such rule is that if you fail to attend a group meeting, one or more other members are assigned to call to find out why you did not attend, and to see if you are having any problems. Just knowing that they will call is an incentive to keep up regular attendance.

Another rule is that all members know each other's phone numbers, and volunteer to receive calls from people in crisis. In order to resign from a group, a member is required to stand up in front of the group and explain why she no longer plans to attend. Then other members get a chance to try to convince her to stay, unless the reason for leaving is valid (e.g., moving away). These rules are listed in the support contracts included in the Plan described in Chapter Eight.

Casual social support outside of a group is also important. As much as possible, try to shop for food with a friend, eat with friends, and exercise with friends. One of the most important factors in happiness is socializing with others. Their influence on you to do the right behaviors is essential to keep on track.

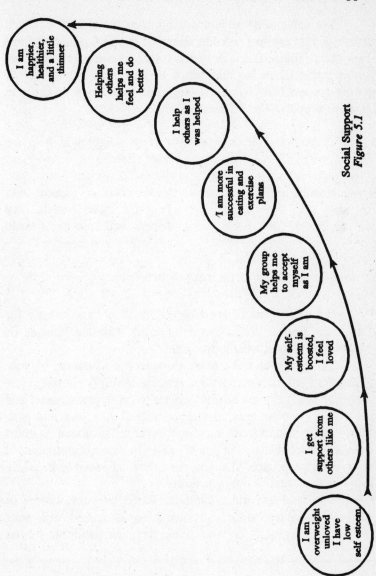

Social Support
Figure 5.1

The value of social support is shown in Figure 5.1. If you are overweight and feel unloved, a support group can help you feel better about yourself, and help control your eating and exercise. Compare this figure with Figure 4.1. The critical difference is seeking support first, rather than trying to lose weight in order to get more support. The difference is this:

- Obese Self Thinking: Losing weight will help me have friends.

- Healthy Self Thinking: Finding social support will help me have friends. My friends will help me manage my eating and exercise.

Picking Your Support Group Carefully

Not all cliques of overweight individuals are suitable for getting the kind of social support needed. Consider friends or associates who have weight problems.

Do they ever criticize or ostracize you because of your appearance? Are they competitive about weight-loss efforts? (*I lost more than you!*) Do you all get together to eat inappropriately and thus help each other give in to temptations? Are your efforts to control eating and exercise sabotaged because friends, in an effort to make you feel better, tell you it's all right that you ate/remained inactive inappropriately? Do you think they may want to keep you from being successful out of jealousy?

One final important question: Based on your success in weight management since you have been associated with your current social group, do you think this association has been helpful?

TYPES OF GROUPS

Some group dieting efforts have been described as rituals with a religious quality.[9] The *sin* is being fat and not controlling eating. Members of the cult worship the god of thinness. Such groups view being fat as a moral problem. Fat members are identified as *overeaters*. In meetings, they *confess* their eating transgressions. This can be damaging to self-esteem if the method of weight management (restrictive dieting) is doomed to produce only short-term losses followed by relapse and regain. Some people who regularly attend this kind of meeting begin to think of themselves as hopeless sinners. This is not good for self-esteem, and leads to a self-fulfilling prophecy: *I am a hopeless sinner in terms of eating control; therefore I might as well give up trying to do better.*

One group well worth considering is Overeaters Anonymous (OA). This is an international non-profit organization providing free self-help groups for compulsive overeaters. It is based on the 12 Steps of Alcoholics Anonymous. These steps can be confusing to the beginner, but they basically cover the following processes:

- *Admitting that your problem is out of control.* As we discussed in Chapter Three, continued failure at weight management has the characteristics of a compulsion, and you can't get out of it all by yourself.

- *Believing that a Power greater than yourself could restore you to sanity.* This Power can be God, support people, or God acting through support people, depending on your religious beliefs or lack of beliefs. Regular attendance at OA meetings may provide the kind of social support described earlier in this chapter.

- *Working with God/support people to rethink and redo your life with respect to food, eating, and relationships.* This corresponds to escaping from your obese self to become your healthy self.

- After entering into recovery, *reaching out to help others who have compulsive eating problems.* This kind of support may be very important in helping maintain your recovery from old patterns.

A survey of OA members showed that those who keep attending lose an average of 24 pounds.[10] This is a good result compared to clinical treatment programs. The survey was not a scientific sample, so it is impossible to say whether everyone who goes to OA has this degree of success. It is probably safe to say that many people get very valuable social support, and are able to boost their self-esteem and lead happier, more productive lives because of OA.

Although the principles of OA are sound, the quality of each group is dependent on the members who attend. Some groups may be dominated by persons who have their own strange ideas about nutrition and exercise, even though OA does not recommend any particular eating or exercise plan. Other groups may be made up of people who are predisposed to sit around and feel sorry for themselves, and to focus on the depressing aspects of having a dependence on food. OA groups are supposed to be uplifting; the 12 Steps provide a way to a better existence. Group members should focus on the positive aspects of growth and recovery. They should recognize that compulsive eating is a physiological reaction to dieting, not a character flaw.[11] If you live in a big city, you will find a large number of OA groups. Shop around until you find one that feels good.

There is another national, low-cost weight management program which meets weekly in groups, Weight Watchers. Weight Watchers provides good nutritional and exercise advice and the group meetings can provide social support, although the level of support may not be as intensive as that described above. If the support is not very profound, you could get together with other members to have an additional weekly group based on the principles of this book.

There are other resources for finding a support group or starting one of your own. You may already have several friends who are willing to meet to follow the suggestions outlined in this book. You might generate some interest at your place of worship, or even at your place of work. You could find a psychotherapist willing to organize a group at her practice. Whatever group you find, it is essential that the group members adhere to the values of the healthy self as listed in Chapter Four, and reject the values of the obese self.

Some may have difficulty obtaining social support. Some may have very low self-esteem, or suffer from depression. This may make reaching out to form or join a group very difficult. Social skills may be limited, making efforts to gather support people unsuccessful. Individuals who have such problems may want to consult a psychotherapist to help relieve depression, and to learn the interpersonal skills needed to become part of a support group. See Appendix A about selecting a weight management clinic which can arrange for such counseling.

Amy

Amy is a 35-year-old school teacher. She has had a weight problem since early childhood. She has never married. She reported binge eating about three times per month. Her writings as part of therapy reflected a profound loneliness and feelings of alienation:

> *I think my parents loved me. I was an only child so I have no way to make a comparison. Both of my parents are rather plump. I may have felt bonded to them since we all shared a weight problem. They certainly never criticized me for my weight, at least not directly.*
>
> *My first memory of rejection due to being fat was in elementary school, like being picked last for kickball teams. I think the kids laughed a little harder when I fell down than for the thin kids. I remember one group who called me and another heavy girl friend the 'fat twins.' They may have called us that only a few times but it really sticks in my memory. I suppose I shouldn't let that kind of thing bother me now.*
>
> *In junior high school I still had the same fat girl friend. When everyone else was getting into dating, I felt safer doing things with her. I worried about being 'queer,' but never had any sexual feelings towards her.*
>
> *During this time, the other kids more or less ignored me. I did very well in school and got some respect from other smart students. I remember finishing ninth grade thinking to myself that I still had never had a date, and I feared that I might never. At this point I was about 50 pounds overweight.*
>
> *In high school I was a nerd book worm. I remember fantasizing that I would be a doctor and that would show the others how good I was compared to them. I guess I really did have some hatred for the 'in' crowd. In college I felt too depressed to do well, but I got a BA in literature. I still find a lot of comfort in reading novels, both modern and classics. Whenever I see a movie about people having fun in college, I know I missed a great deal by being a loner.*
>
> *A thin classmate in college asked me if I overate. She was a compulsive overeater and convinced me to go to an Overeaters*

Anonymous meeting. At the OA meetings, I realized there were a lot of others suffering from feelings of guilt, shame and loneliness because of being unable to control eating. I developed some friendships there, and went to some OA parties where I really had fun in a social setting for the first time in my life. I never got a sponsor, and my attendance is sporadic, but I maintain a few friends from OA. We go out together and share feelings. I think it has helped me to reduce my temptation to binge.

Progress: Amy is being encouraged to continue interacting in small groups to get out her feelings of depression caused by a lifetime of social isolation. She is beginning to see how her eating problem was related to loneliness. She also appreciates using the group to 'police' her tendency to over- or under-eat.

THE BOTTOM LINE:

- Social support boosts self-esteem.

- Social support persons can give advice.

- Social support can help you feel accepted and normal.

- Success requires careful selection of social support.

- You need social support to help avoid over- and under-eating.

Awareness Exercises

1. Have you ever been in a group which provided the kind of support discussed in this chapter? Describe the group and how it felt to be a member.

    _____

    _____

    _____

    _____

    Most people's happiest memories are of times when they were sharing with others. More effort should be put on small groups getting together through clubs and places of worship. Too many of us live lives of detachment and independence.

2. When you were a child, did your family provide good social support? Describe the good and bad aspects of the support you got from your family.

    _____

    _____

    _____

    The nuclear family is probably not as good for providing social support as was the extended family system of previous generations. Now, even the nuclear family structure of our society is breaking up.

3.   Do you think your parents had a particularly good or bad
      influence on your self-esteem and problems with eating
      control? Describe:

      _____

      _____

      _____

      _____

*Many parents seem to be over- or under-involved with
their female children's eating and appearance. Parental
over-involvement often leads to psychological problems
relating to food and eating disorders. But under-
involvement can allow poor nutritional habits to become
ingrained in the children.*

4.   Do you think you are a worthwhile enough person to get
      the kind of in-depth support described?

      _____

      _____

      _____

*Often patients say "I'm probably just wasting your time."
Their self-esteem is so low they feel they don't deserve
help. A good support group can help individuals realize
that they are valuable.*

5. If you feel unworthy, or feel you wouldn't belong in a group, you may need to be in a group in order to work on having a better opinion of yourself. Discuss:

_____

_____

_____

_____

If our patients say that they feel uncomfortable in groups, we try especially hard to prepare them to interact in a group and to make sure they join one. We do this because of our conviction that happiness and fulfillment in life are very difficult to achieve if a person remains socially isolated.

6.   Write down the names of people who would support you. Connect the dots between each name and the kinds of support each person gives you.

                                                     O   helps me through crises

1._____O   O   helpful advice

2._____O   O   encouragement

3._____O   O   shares experiences

4._____O   O   shares emotions

5._____O   O confronts me with truth

6._____O   O   gives me feedback

                                                     O makes me feel normal

                                                   O boosts my self-esteem

If you are fortunate and have a lot of support, this will look like the web of a spider on drugs. If you have few lines, then follow the instructions in Chapter Eight carefully.

6

BECOMING AN EXERCISE ENTHUSIAST

About one hundred years ago, many Americans were farmers. Farming was not so easy back then. You couldn't plow a field riding in air-conditioned comfort with a four-speaker sound system. Farmers' wives had to chop wood, maintain a garden, do laundry and clean house without modern conveniences. Farming is still not the easiest profession. However, in the last century, farmers did the equivalent of ten miles of jogging every day to run their farms; their wives put in the equivalent of about seven miles of jogging every day.

There are still parts of the world where humans live in primitive conditions. Deep in the rain forest of Peru, a man may spend all day running after a monkey, trying to fell it from the tree tops with a blow-gun loaded with poison darts.[1] After about 5 miles of running, and after climbing about ten 100-foot trees, the native is able to make the final kill, and get about 5 pounds of lean meat. How much effort did you expend the last time you bought a bag of potato chips? (Note: A one-pound bag of potato chips has 2600 calories. Five pounds of lean monkey has about 2800 calories.)

These illustrations tell us that if we want to control obesity, we need to change our thinking about exercise. From a species which spent a good deal of time and energy in getting enough food to eat, we have become such clever city dwellers that large quantities of calories can be obtained without any effort at all. Now, we are not suggesting that people should have to exercise to get food. However, in the face of easily obtainable calories, we need to add exercise to our sedentary lifestyles so that our bodies have a chance to achieve an energy balance without storing up fat reserves.

Many hold the belief that overweight people are lazy. It is true that they tend to exercise less than thin people. However, this is not due to any fault of character. We think it is due to lack of knowledge about how to become enthusiastic about exercise. Due to the vicious cycles of dieting and loss of eating control described in Chapter Three, overweight people end up carrying around excess weight and losing physical fitness. This makes them more tired, leading to another vicious cycle in terms of lowered energy.

Energy Sappers

A common complaint among many Americans is that they feel tired during the day. Unless you have a medical problem, the reasons for feeling tired could be:

- not enough sleep
- not enough exercise
- poor nutrition
- too much stress
- too many poisons in the body (alcohol and drugs)

A gentleman came to us complaining of fatigue in the afternoon. He had gone to his doctor, who gave him a thorough check-up, which found nothing unusual. The doctor gave him a prescription for a stimulant drug so that he could have more pep in the P.M. The drug worked. But was that the best solution? We discovered that this man was eating no breakfast except coffee, had a meal replacement drink for lunch to help control his minor weight problem, and did not exercise. We advised him to eat a sensible breakfast and lunch, and to take a long walk every day. This man now has plenty of energy and can just say *No* to drugs.

One of the authors of this book, (GKG), before he became a health psychologist, was an engineer with a rather boring job. His routine included coffee and sweet rolls for breakfast, and enough coffee during the day to stay awake. He was asthmatic as a child, and never exercised. Often, he would find himself nodding off at his desk. This was a very uncomfortable feeling. It is awful to have a strong desire to lie down on a cozy bed but be forced to stay put at a desk trying to focus your brain on complex mathematics. This was at age 23. Now, 22 years later, with proper nutrition and regular aerobic exercise, this person rarely feels tired during the day. He has more energy in middle age than during what should have been his roaring twenties.

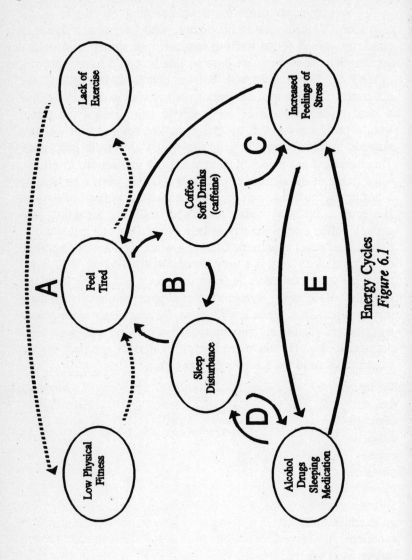

Energy Cycles
Figure 6.1

Many factors work together to sap the energy individuals need to be active and to feel good, as shown in the model of energy cycles (Figure 6.1). Start in the box labelled, *Feel Tired*. If you feel tired, you are unlikely to exercise. This lack of exercise leads to low physical fitness, which is the ability of the body to metabolize oxygen in order to perform work. If ability to perform work is low, the chores you must do every day will make you feel tired, thus completing this vicious cycle of inactivity and fatigue, which is labelled *A*.

If you feel tired, you may turn to caffeine for relief. Caffeine stimulates the central nervous system, increases feelings of stress, increases metabolism, and causes an increase in muscle tension. These activities deplete your energy, which can make you feel tired, completing vicious cycle *C*. Caffeine can disrupt a good night's sleep, even if you are not aware of it. Needless to say, if the depth and quality of your sleep are limited by caffeine, you will tend to feel more tired during your waking hours. This is depicted in vicious cycle *B*.

Chronic use of caffeine, lack of quality sleep, and lack of the stress-reducing effects of exercise (see below) can often drive a person to use alcohol, drugs, or sleeping medications to calm down and to get better sleep. This may work for a short time, but the long-term effects of taking chemicals to promote sleep and to feel calm are worse sleep, and more feelings of stress. This is depicted as cycle *D*. If you continue to turn to alcohol or other drugs to solve sleep and stress problems, you may end up in vicious cycle *E*, which is otherwise known as *alcoholism* or *chemical dependence*. How do you break free of these vicious cycles? Exercise is one way. If you are overweight, and see yourself caught up in any of these cycles, your task is to develop an exercise habit which will build up your fitness level, give you more energy, help you cut down on coffee, alcohol or other drugs, reduce your feelings of stress, and get a good night's sleep.

Living Without Dieting

Here are our recommendations for breaking free of these energy-sapping cycles:

- Exercise by following the program described in Chapter Eight.

- Eat according to the guidelines in Chapter Eight.

- Reduce coffee consumption gradually to no more than 1 cup per day, and no coffee after 4 p.m. Gradual reduction may be required to avoid headaches. Try drinking one less cup per day each week until you are down to one cup per day or none.

- Reduce or eliminate use of alcohol. No more than one drink per day. A drink is defined as 12 ounces of beer, 3 ounces of wine, or 1.5 ounces of liquor.

- Use no sleeping medications, unless prescribed by your physician. Talk to your physician about getting off drugs.

- Quit all uses of tobacco.

The key to becoming an enthusiastic exerciser is energy. If you don't feel energetic, you won't develop and maintain an exercise habit. Our approach to weight control is not self-punishment, but self-enjoyment. People who feel energetic want to exercise. They look forward to it. They feel frustrated if they can't exercise. They enjoy exercise so much that they need no willpower to exercise regularly. You can be like them.

The ways to develop an unshakable motivation to exercise regularly include: learning to enjoy exercise, changing your beliefs and attitudes about exercise, learning to recognize and eliminate excuses not to exercise, increasing awareness of your exercise behavior, controlling your exercise environment, and using visualization to experience the unseen effects of exercise. Sounds like a lot, doesn't it? But if taken one day at a time, in a step-by-step fashion, you can achieve the desired results.

Learning to Enjoy Exercise

Did you hate physical education classes? Did you always get P.E. class early in the morning so that you felt sweaty and unkempt during the rest of the day? Was exercise used as a punishment for not doing enough or for being late? The cruelty of many P.E. programs is well-known. And if you were overweight during your school years, multiply the pain by 10. After experiences like those, it may be difficult to develop a positive attitude toward vigorous exercise. If you see yourself as being caught up in the energy cycles discussed above, you can begin to understand that not exercising is part of a vicious cycle. The more you don't exercise, the more fatigued you become, and the more you desire inactivity. How do you learn to enjoy that which seems horrendous? Little by little.

We hope you are able to walk. If not, you will need to consult with your physician and a physical therapist to determine if there is a possibility of getting exercise in some other way, such as using an exercise bicycle designed for the arms. But let's assume you can walk. Let's assume you can walk around the block. That is all you need to get started. All you have to do is follow these two rules:

1. Exercise at an intensity (or speed) and duration that feel invigorating but not strenuous. In other words, go as fast and long as you can without discomfort.

2.   Never give up.
        (Unless your physician tells you to stop. See
        valid excuses, below).

We have found that if overweight individuals follow these two rules using the walking program described in Chapter Eight, they can learn to enjoy exercise and make it a life-long habit. It could also be called a *long-life* habit, since regular exercise seems to be related to longevity.

In one of our research projects, we taught overweight adults how to enjoy walking. They kept records on their exercise and how they felt during and after exercise. After one year, we analyzed these records. We found that 65 percent were still doing healthful exercise. The records also showed that almost everyone reported feeling *good* or *excellent*, both during and after each exercise experience. The exercise plan we used in this research formed the basis of the plan included in this book. It was designed after the ideas of Dr. John Greist, a psychiatrist who pioneered the use of exercise in the treatment of depression.[2]

We like to call exercise sessions *experiences* because we feel it is important to focus on all the pleasurable experiences involved in exercise. During a walk, for example, you can experience the rhythmic actions of your muscles and lungs, the sight, sound and smell sensations of your walking path, the thoughts that come to you as you spend some time alone in a natural setting. Yes, walking can be a form of recreation. Here is how to think about exercise: *I deserve to enjoy exercise regularly. It also helps me control excess body fat.*

Changing Your Thinking About Exercise

You can change your thinking about exercise by learning how to do it so that it is enjoyable. But it is also helpful to fill your mind with information about the benefits of exercise to keep you motivated. In our research, we have found that most of the overweight people who learn to enjoy exercise make it a lasting habit. But others stop, even though they enjoyed exercise. The reason most of them quit seems to be due to what could be called *life stress*. The life stressors include divorce, job changes, moving to another house, and other events which had nothing to do with whether they should exercise or not. Apparently, under stress, exercise is edged out by other concerns, even though these individuals know that exercise is good for reducing feelings of stress.

In order to make exercise more important, it may be necessary to fill the brain with all kinds of facts about the wonderful effects of exercise. Often it seems that when we have to make a decision, there are two debate teams challenging each other in our head. The team that wins is the one with the most persuasive argument based on the most facts. If you are filled with facts in favor of exercise when life stressors occur, your pro-exercise debate team can win. It is said, *It's all right to argue with yourself as long as you don't lose to the side that's against you.*

So let's fill up your brain with the facts about exercise.

HEALTH BENEFITS:

- Heart muscle is made stronger and more efficient
- Helps reduce blood pressure
- Reduces resting heart rate
- More oxygen gets to cells
- Good cholesterol is increased
- Fat deposits on body are reduced
- Reduces risk of having heart attack
- Elasticity of arteries is increased
- Reduces risk of osteoporosis (brittle bones)
- Prevents reductions in metabolism caused by eating less
- Slows down the aging process

- Improves lung efficiency
- Tones up muscles
- Improves sleep

PSYCHOLOGICAL BENEFITS:

- Reduces uncomfortable reactions to stress
- Helps you feel good and fight depression
- Makes you feel more energetic
- Improves self-esteem
- Improves appearance, makes you thinner
- Gives you an enjoyable experience
- Keeps your mind alert as you age
- Helps keep your physical reactions quick as you age
- Some say it makes you sexier and improves sex

It might also be motivational to look at the other side of the coin, or the

DISADVANTAGES OF NOT EXERCISING:

- Makes you more likely to get dread diseases
- Makes you tired
- Makes you age more quickly
- Makes you fatter

Question: When you are older, do you want to be thought of as someone who needs to take a nap, or someone who has the vitality and energy to participate fully in enjoyable recreational activities? Exercise is the key. As the shoe people say, *Just do it*. And as we say, *Just enjoy it*.

Mind Control

Often, when we are deciding whether to do something, we weigh the pros and cons of the behavior in our minds. We think of the advantages and disadvantages of each course of action, as listed above. Suppose you have thought about the advantages of exercising. Suppose you are just about to put on your walking shoes and take an enjoyable walk. But then something strange happens in your mind. From somewhere, deep in your subconscious, comes a jumble of distorted thinking. Soon these thoughts become clearer, and you realize that you are dealing with your less desirable side. Remember in the movie cartoons when the main character has an angel on one shoulder and a devil on the other, and they are trying to persuade him to do the right and wrong thing? Up from the depths of your mind come the excuse thoughts. An excuse thought is a reason which you have created to *justify* not exercising.

A typical excuse thought goes like this: *I should exercise today, but there is this show on television I want to see, and I can always exercise tomorrow instead.* Presto! You have a reason for not exercising. If you have enough excuse thoughts in your head, you can come up with reasons not to do a lot. Let's face it. Most people do not behave in an ideal fashion. There is a big difference between what we know we should do and what we actually do. Religions explain this using the concept of sin. Whether or not you believe in the concept of sin, you probably recognize excuse thoughts.

Here is another secret of motivation: *Self control is running out of excuses not to do the right thing.*

Here is how this secret can be applied to help you become an enthusiastic and regular exerciser. First, identify all the excuse thoughts you may have regarding exercise. Then come up with a counter argument for each one. After developing a counter argument for an excuse thought, you cannot fool yourself again.

EXCUSE THOUGHTS FOR NOT EXERCISING

EXCUSE:	COUNTER ARGUMENT:
I don't have enough time.	Regular exercise requires only about 5 percent of your waking hours. If you can't fit that into your schedule, your life is probably very stressful and you really need exercise badly to help unwind. Having regular exercise helps in coping with stress.
I'm too tired to exercise.	Many people who feel exhausted at the end of the day feel refreshed when they exercise in the evening. Some people who hate to get up early find that an early morning workout gives them more energy to start their day.
Exercise is too boring.	If exercise is done regularly, 3 to 4 times per week, for 30+ minutes each time, exercise will be pleasurable. If not, ride an exercise bike in front of a TV or while reading. Walking with friends is fun. Walk a dog.
Exercise makes me sore.	If you gradually increase your exercise, you will have little soreness. After a few weeks, any soreness will disappear and exercise will feel good.

EXCUSE:	**COUNTER ARGUMENT:**
As a housewife with kids, I can't leave home.	Get an exercise bike. Go for a walk with your kids. Form a babysitting co-op.
(For women) Exercise will make me look like a man.	Most of the top female TV and movie stars do a lot of exercise. Fitness is definitely *in* for women.
Exercise causes injuries.	If you follow a gradual approach, the probability of injury is minimal. Your chances of developing diseases caused by a lack of exercise are much greater. Walking is the safest form of exercise.
Exercise makes me too tired.	Regular exercise will give you more energy.
I'm too old to exercise.	You are never too old to benefit from regular exercise. Brisk walking is the perfect exercise for all ages. (See a physician first.)
I'm too fat to exercise.	Exercise is one of the most important parts of a weight control program. Exercise is highly correlated to success in keeping weight off.

EXCUSE:	COUNTER ARGUMENT:
I have too many personal problems to begin an exercise program.	Regular exercise is a good way to help you handle the mental and physical stress of life. It is relaxing and keeps your body and mind healthy.
I'm depressed. I don't want to do anything.	Regular exercise can be very good to help you feel less depressed.
I feel self-conscious exercising in front of other people.	Others will be envious of you in your new healthful exercise program. Have a T-shirt made which says *Remodeling Underway* or *What's So Funny, Thinso?* This will help you communicate to others in a way that will make you feel less self-conscious.
I get asthma when I exercise.	Many people can successfully prevent exercise-induced asthma with medication. See your physician.

Now list some of your own excuse thoughts:

Excuse Thoughts   **Counter Arguments**

_____   _____

_____   _____

_____   _____

_____   _____

_____   _____

Very good. You may want to copy these excuse thoughts and their counter arguments and post them on the wall in your house for repeated readings.

You may think we are being too tough by taking away all excuses not to exercise. Well, we are not cruel. We are now going to give to you some excuses for not exercising. These are the only valid excuses that we have discovered. If you discover any others, be sure to write us. Here are the valid excuses:

VALID EXCUSES NOT TO EXERCISE

1. A licensed physician has told you not to exercise. (Get a second opinion.)

2. Your area is under a tornado or hurricane warning.

3. Flood waters around your house are above one foot in depth.

4.   A madman is holding you at gunpoint and will shoot if you move.

5.   You feel faint, nauseous, have a migraine, a fever, or any other condition which requires medical attention.

More Mind Control: Total Awareness

In order to develop the habit, you will need to be totally aware of your exercise behavior. One way to do this is to keep careful records of your exercise sessions, and of the times when you did not exercise as planned. Most people can't accurately remember whether they did or did not exercise on any particular day a week ago. If you write down your exercise experiences you will be aware of how frequently you are exercising, how long you exercised, and how you felt during and after exercise. You can see your progress over a long period of time.

You can also make a note of the times you didn't exercise as planned, and why you didn't. Was your excuse valid or invalid? What could you do to prevent this barrier to exercise from occurring again?   Self-monitoring forms for recording your exercise experiences are included in Chapter Eight.

If you faithfully record your exercise on these forms, you will maintain a high level of awareness about your habit formation. You will be less able to fool yourself about whether you are making progress or regress. We sum up this section with another secret of motivation:

Success in weight-loss is highly correlated with faithful self-monitoring. People who keep records are more likely to succeed. So do it.

Stimulus Control of Exercise

Much of our behavior is triggered by external factors or events, which psychologists call *stimuli*. If you want to trigger good behavior, such as exercising, you can set up your environment so that exercise becomes more likely. Here are some examples:

- Set aside a particular time for exercise so that it becomes a part of your schedule. This way a certain time can be a trigger for exercise, instead of you trying to *fit* exercise into random periods of spare time. Make exercise a priority, as important as sleeping and eating.

- Make sure your exercise clothes and equipment are ready and visible to you, so that you can immediately get ready for exercise before a dreaded excuse thought gets hold of your better intentions.

- Arrange to exercise with one or more people. Then they can trigger you to exercise.

- Execute a contract with family members, friends, and/or coworkers which says that you will get some reward if you stick to your exercise plan. This can be highly motivational since most people want to look good to others.

- Subscribe to a walking or exercise magazine which is filled with informational and motivational material. Then, every month you will receive a reminder that you are an enthusiastic exerciser. See Appendix B for examples.

- Join a fitness club. But beware. Many people sign up for years of membership in such clubs when they are highly motivated and influenced by the gorgeous salespeople and fancy equipment. But about 90 percent fail to keep using the club, because it becomes too much trouble to go there when motivation is lower. Think carefully about the advantages of exercising on your own before forking over the money to a club. Do you know for certain that you will use it regularly for a long time?

You can see that stimulus control means that you do something now which changes future stimuli in a way that makes exercise more likely. Consider the cases of Rose and Jane, who both want to increase their exercise in order to control excess body fat:

Rose: *I always tell myself Friday night that I am going to get up early Saturday morning at sunrise and walk for about an hour. It would be so lovely to walk at that time when there is no traffic and I can be alone with the birds and squirrels. But I usually wake up at 7 a.m. and it feels so good just to lie in bed for another two hours. So that's what I do. Then I feel guilty about not exercising, and I know guilt is a negative emotion which probably hurts my self-control of eating during the day.*

Jane: *I like to walk on Saturday morning as the sun comes up. It is so peaceful. So on Friday night, I set my alarm for about half an hour before I plan to get out of bed. I also program my coffee maker to have fresh coffee ready for me when I get up. I arrange all my exercise clothes and shoes on the chair before going to bed. The next morning, I get out of bed, put on my exercise outfit and have a cup of coffee. The game I play with myself is that I don't decide whether to exercise or not until after coffee. After coffee, with my walking shoes on, I almost always decide to go out to exercise.*

What is Rose's mistake? She didn't arrange to have stimuli in the morning to motivate her to exercise. Another error was that she allowed herself to make a decision whether to exercise or not while she was still snug in bed. They say don't make a decision to buy a car while you are at the dealer because there is too much sales pressure there. Likewise, don't decide to forgo exercise when you are half asleep.

If you are tired in the afternoon or evening, don't decide to skip exercise. Get your exercise gear on, and walk around the block once or twice. If you still feel terrible, then you can choose to stop. But most of the time you will feel better, finish your walk, and feel energetic and proud when you finish. For individuals who like to listen to cassette tapes while walking or jogging, one author (JPF) recommends renting them from *Books on Tape, Inc.*, or *Recorded Books, Inc.* (Addresses and telephone numbers are in Appendix B.) Over the past year, while jogging, he has listened to the complete versions of *Pride and Prejudice, David Copperfield, Great Expectations, Tess of the D'Urbervilles, Wuthering Heights, Crime and Punishment, Don Quixote, The Adventures of Tom Sawyer, The Adventures of Huckleberry Finn*, and *Brideshead Revisited*, among others. He especially recommends the *Books on Tape, Inc.* version of Larry McMurtry's *Lonesome Dove*, and *Anything for Billy*, and the *Recorded Books, Inc.* version of Charles Dickens' *A Tale of Two Cities*. There are many books one can listen to while exercising.

Visualization

In order to realize a goal, have a clear picture of it in your head. Not just a picture of the benefits of achieving the goal, but a picture of the good feelings you will have about your accomplishment. We have already talked about some of the psychological and health benefits of exercise. In this section we present some mental exercises to help you focus on the emotional aspects of exercise benefits.

Here are two poems that depict both negative and positive visualization:

Visualization for Couch Potatoes

I sit quietly,
As video shadows
Move across my vision,
Relentlessly hawking
The fat and sweet morsels
Of temptation better left eschewed
Than eaten.

Cells of fat
Assiduously absorb and store
The calories which,
For want of movement,
Are fated to my thighs,
My middle, my rear,
My guilt.

Slowly and inexorably,
With each passing minute,
I grow older, more stale.
Decay and disease
Are my destiny,
Fatigue and frustration
My future.

By G. Ken Goodrick and Phyllis Heyder-O'Donnell

Now, in a more positive vein, here is a

Visualization for Exercisers

Fresh air greets my face
As I jog, or walk at a fast pace
Making oxygen flow freely
Into my lungs, blood, and cells.
Energizing my muscles
Which rhythmically carry me forward
To my firmer self.

Walking free with arms and body
Abandoned to the thrill
Of luxurious movement
I fully experience my animal nature.
My instinctive quest!

By G. Ken Goodrick and Phyllis Heyder-O'Donnell

If you have inspirational material, please send it to us so that we may include it in future editions.

Final Thoughts on Exercise

Suppose you owned a pedigreed descendent of Rin Tin Tin, the wonder dog of Hollywood fame. Would you keep it in a cage so small that exercise was impossible? Of course not. You would arrange for this dog to have a large yard in which to run. Everyone knows that animals need and enjoy exercise. Don't keep yourself in a cage.

Speaking of animals, research has shown that rats put on diets with yo-yo weight fluctuations increase their preference for high-fat foods.[3] This preference may be prevented with exercise.[4] Thus exercise may help in appetite control by reducing the cravings for high-fat foods.

Sandra

Sandra is a 40-year-old store manager who has had a weight problem since early adolescence. She told us that she suffered from chronic fatigue and that was why she couldn't exercise. Her physician reported that there was no apparent medical condition causing fatigue. This is what she wrote about her struggle with exercise:

My earliest memories about exercise are that I used to stay home a lot when I was young and watch TV. No one in my family exercised or thought that I should. I remember staying on the sidelines during games at recess since I didn't feel like running.

In junior high school I became very self-conscious of my appearance- I guess everybody did- although I wasn't very overweight then, maybe 20 or 30 pounds. I hated P.E. mainly because it required me to exercise but also because it was so hard to look good after sweating and hurrying to get made up in a hot locker room. Also I noticed that I looked like kind of a blob compared to most of the other girls who were thin and had more breast development than I did.

In high school there was no P.E. requirement so I took music classes as electives. Maybe I was identifying with large opera stars. I remember having trouble staying awake in class. I felt this was due to rapid growth during my teen years. I usually feel most comfortable relaxing, and have taken naps several times a week since childhood. I gained another 20 pounds in high school, probably due to me and my friends getting heavily into pizza.

When I went to college in the 70's the fitness craze was just beginning. I actually bought a sweat suit and started walking at night around the campus. Back then I used to think that sweating helped in weight control. The first week my thighs got really sore, and a man surprised me coming around a corner. I remember going back to my dorm thinking that exercise wasn't worth the effort, and thinking it would be safer just to do some calisthenics in my room.

Sometime later I started walking with a friend. She went much faster than I wanted to. I got a pain in my ankle which the doctor said might be due to too much weight. I had been dieting off and on for years, but it didn't seem to help except to drop 10 pounds for a few weeks.

After I got my first job, I joined an exercise club which was fun because they had all kinds of equipment, swimming pool, sauna and good-looking instructors. After a while though it seemed that everyone there belonged to a clique of thin athletes. After two months of regular attendance at the club, I didn't notice much change in my appearance, although I did feel more energetic and relaxed. Then I had to go on some business trips, and I remember getting the flu after one of the trips. I guess this broke my exercise habit because I never did get back to the club except for a few times.

I felt guilty about not exercising, partly because I didn't get my money's worth from the club's membership fee. I haven't been able to figure out why I never got back into regular exercise even though I enjoyed it and I know I feel better when I do it. Maybe I can't stick to exercise for the same reason I can't stick to a diet-lack of willpower.

Progress: Sandra is beginning to think about exercise in a way that will make it a higher priority in her life. The group members are keeping track of her progress. She calls a group member whenever she feels tempted to skip an exercise session. She appreciates the gradual, self-regulated approach to exercise, and realizes that she probably was overdoing exercise most of the time in her past. She now knows that her fatigue is caused by lack of exercise.

THE BOTTOM LINE:

● Exercise is mandatory for successful weight management and health.

● It is also mandatory that exercise be enjoyable.

Awareness Exercises

1. Describe your experiences with vigorous exercise from childhood on.

    _____

    _____

    _____

    Not many people were lucky enough to have parents who were exercise enthusiasts and who engendered a love for sports and fitness in their children. Many individuals who are now middle-aged had parents who were enjoying the sedentary lifestyle made possible by modern industrial techniques.

2. If you are not currently exercising, what are the barriers within yourself?

    _____

    _____

    _____

    Do you really hate exercise? Have you ever tried a very gradual approach? Do you consider exercise to be a punishment for being too fat? Do you feel silly or embarrassed to exercise in public?

3.   Are there any barriers outside of yourself which prevent your exercising?

_____

_____

_____

_____

Be active in finding safe places to walk. Make an exercise place in your home.

4.   You believe that people think you are lazy because of your weight problem. But you also feel self-conscious exercising in public. How can you resolve these two thoughts?

_____

_____

_____

_____

Why should you be concerned with what others may be thinking? It is only important that you are doing the right thing to improve yourself. Why should you let thin people control your exercise behavior?

5. Visualize how your life will be different when you become fit with regular exercise. What do you have to look forward to?

_____

_____

_____

_____

Do you know any older persons who exercise regularly? Do you want to be like the little old lady who jogged 6 miles a day at age 80? Do you think she was able to enjoy life more than the average 80-year-old?

7

HOW TO BECOME A LOW-FAT EATER

...Give us nothing but vegetables to eat and water to drink. Then compare our appearance with that of the young men who eat the royal food, and treat your servants in accordance with what you see. So he agreed to this and tested them for ten days.

At the end of ten days they looked healthier and better nourished than any of the young men who ate the royal food. So the guard took away their choice food and the wine they were to drink and gave them vegetables instead.[1]

A few moments ago, the co-author (GKG) who wrote this sentence was out wandering about the medical center where he is employed. He was wondering how to begin this chapter on eating. As he approached a snack shop, he decided to go in and buy a chocolate bar. According to the label, this 1.45-ounce bar contained:

14 grams of fat
18 grams of sugar (simple carbohydrate)
2 grams of carbohydrates
5 grams of protein
230 calories

Fat has 9 calories per gram, carbohydrates and protein each have 4 calories per gram. Thus, this bar was 54.8 percent fat and 31 percent sugar in terms of total calories. This explains why it tasted so good.

Where does this guy who wrote this chapter get the nerve to tell the reader that he just enjoyed what many overweight people consider to be their number one nemesis? Here is how: He has discovered the secret of how to eat all the high-fat food he wants and still keep his weight under control! Does this sound like a miracle? Do you have visions of eating large quantities of fried foods, cakes, cookies, pies, chips, dips, and eclairs without gaining excess body fat?

Sorry. You can't eat large quantities of high-fat foods and control your weight. So how does this so-called secret work? Read the last paragraph again. It says he eats all the high-fat food he wants. The secret is in changing how much you want. That is what this chapter is about.

Our Changing Food Environment

Remember the Peruvian native who spent all day chasing after some monkey meat? He has the proper balance of good exercise and low-fat eating. He needs no willpower to control his weight. Obesity doesn't even occur in his village. But poor modern man. High-fat foods are everywhere. And inexpensive. A century ago, Americans used to spend up to 40 percent of their family budget on food. Now food only costs us about 15 percent of our income (Yes, there are some poor people in our country who spend more than that on food, but we are talking averages.)

Not only is food easier to obtain and afford, it is also too high in fat. The average American diet is 37 percent fat. Why is this? In large part it is due to the practices of the food industry. Take chickens for example. They used to run around the farmyard eating corn. Now, some chicken farms have massive buildings which each hold 10,000 chickens. These birds live in little cages. One conveyor belt runs by their cage with food. Another belt runs under the cage to remove chicken droppings. You can imagine that such chickens are not in a state of peak physical condition.

When you buy one of these chickens at the store, examine it closely. You may see clumps of yellow fat attached to the muscle. Depending on the quality of your store, there may also be hunks of yellow fat hidden under the meat. These chickens, if left to live longer, may develop obesity and heart disease. However, they are sacrificed at a young age, so that we humans may eat their fat and become obese and get heart disease.

What about beef? When you eat beef, are you eating the fit muscle of a proud animal which was recently roaming the range? Or are you eating the fatty muscle of an emasculated creature which has been given hormones and kept penned-in prior to slaughter to add the desired marbling of fat?

What about chips? There is a brand of potato chips which claims on the bag that the chips are simply *fried slices of potato, one of nature's nutritious foods*. There are more words designed to make the purchaser of these chips feel good about the nutritional value of chips. You can calculate the nutrition of potato chips from the information printed on the package. In terms of calories, a baked potato has about 20 calories per ounce. Potato chips are made out of potatoes and fat, and have about 160 calories per ounce. You can conclude that in terms of calories, potato chips are seven parts fat and one part potato.

We wondered about all this. We wrote to the manufacturer of these chips with some recommendations. We pointed out that the wording on the package suggested that potato chips were nutritious and that eating them was a good idea. We felt this was misleading, since adding so much fat to potatoes is not nutritionally advisable. In fact, we suggested that to be perfectly honest, their product should be called *Fat Chips*, in order to reflect the main ingredient.

The response we got suggested that we mind our own business. Now, we are not saying that the food industry is the enemy. They are not trying to force fat down our throats to make us all obese. They are trying to make money. A good way to make money is to sell products which people want. Many people want high-fat foods. High-fat foods are tasty.

But there is a growing number of people who are demanding lower-fat foods. The food industry is trying to make changes. You can get *light* corn and potato chips which are made with less fat. (We still don't recommend them.) You can get baked rather than fried corn tortillas (good idea). You can get *light* beef from special breeds of cattle which have been fed a good diet with adequate exercise. You can buy reduced fat frankfurters if you really must have a frankfurter. You can go to a salad bar at a fast food hamburger restaurant.

You can now get no-fat yogurt and cottage cheese. There is fat-free and sugar-free frozen yogurt which actually is very good. There are fat-free sweet rolls and pound cake. Fat substitutes made from proteins are the new rage. So there is hope. With the new modern food technology, we are beginning to solve some of the problems of the old food technology.

Our food environment may actually be losing some of its fat. But Americans, especially our children, are still getting fatter and fatter, year by year. There are still entire aisles in the supermarket which contain only high sugar and high-fat items, such as the soft-drink/chips aisle, or the ice cream/frozen pies and cakes section. Yes, it is still too easy to eat high-fat foods.

Fat and Energy

In Chapter Six we talked about the importance of feeling energetic. You are more likely to get needed exercise if you feel energetic. What should you eat to maintain a high energy level? Foods with lots of energy? Fat has 2.5 times more energy in terms of calories per ounce than does protein or carbohydrate. Therefore you should eat fat for energy, right? Wrong.

We once found a product sold at a health food store which was labelled *Energy Drink*. It claimed to give you *2.5 times as much energy as protein*. This energy drink consisted of vegetable oil and some vitamin E. It is true that this drink would give you more energy than protein, but in terms of calories, not pep.

In fact, high-fat foods may sap your feelings of energy. Research with animals shows that when fed a high energy density (high in fat) diet, they will become less active and sleep more.[2] Most humans do not want to get up and run around after consuming large amounts of pizza.

Thus, eating high-fat foods may be a double-whammy. Not only do you get more calories from fat which can lead to obesity, but you are also less likely to exercise. This can lead to the vicious cycles shown in Figure 7.1. Most people hate to feel tired. A good motivation to become a low-fat eater is to focus on how much more energetic we feel after eating wisely.

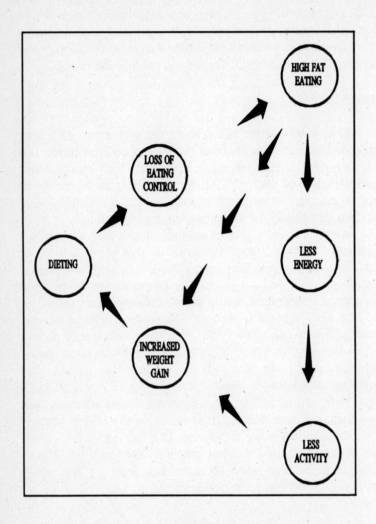

Vicious Cycles Related to High-Fat Eating
Figure 7.1

Reducing Desire for High-Fat Foods

Do you love to eat high-fat foods? Most people do. They are enjoyable because we are designed to go after the high-calorie opportunities to eat. We do this because our appetites are adjusted to earlier times when calories were scarce. Now that our food environment consists of many high-fat opportunities, we have the same problem as the bearded tits. So what can we do? One approach is to do things which will reduce cravings.

Stop Dieting

One of the most important things to do to gain control over your eating is to stop dieting. In Chapter Three we pointed out that dieting can lead to serious self-control problems in eating, including binging and purging. Some people stick to a rigorous schedule of meal replacements for breakfast and lunch. At dinnertime they will have half a grapefruit, and possibly half a piece of dry toast. Then at 10 p.m. they will have three servings of cheesecake for a snack.

Forget self-starvation. To curb cravings, eat three meals a day, with two between-meal snacks. The eating plan included in Chapter Eight shows you what to eat. The idea is that sensible eating spread out over the day stabilizes your blood sugar so that hunger never gets to be much of a problem.

Sensible eating means eating according to the recommendations of the Surgeon General, the American Heart Association, and the American Cancer Society. Fortunately, these organizations agree on what's good for us. Isn't it nice to know that what we need to eat to control our excess body fat is also good for reducing the risk of heart disease and cancer? These eating recommendations also should help increase feelings of energy and prevent constipation.

As recommended by the above groups, we need to eat more complex carbohydrates and less protein and fat. Complex carbohydrates are metabolized more slowly than simple ones, so that blood sugar level and appetite tend to be more stable. If you eat according to the plan described in Chapter Eight, you will get the correct balance of nutrients.

Easy Does It

If you have been a high-fat eater most of your life, you will not want to shock your system by suddenly switching to healthful eating. It is also difficult to make big changes in life-long habits. One alternative is gradually to increase the number of *low-fat* eating days that you have each week. A low-fat eating day is one in which everything you eat is relatively low in fat.

There is another reason for gradual change. If you try to eat only low-fat foods immediately, you are likely to have a lapse back to one of your old favorites, like grandma's fried chicken. You will then feel like a failure. So our plan recommends that you start off having low-fat *meals*. Then you can have a low-fat day. As you progress, you can slowly increase the number of low-fat *days* each month. This allows you to have some mistakes without feeling like a failure. Remember: *feelings of failure facilitate failure*.

We know that some of you may be telling yourself, *This gradual change approach is for wimps. I am going to start eating only low-fat foods immediately*. Well, good luck to you. But be warned. Remember the finger puzzle in Chapter One. If you are over-motivated you may be setting yourself up for under-achievement. Cut yourself some slack. Our plan is designed to be an enjoyable way to low-fat eating. And if a plan is enjoyable, the likelihood of relapse due to negative emotions is minimized.

As discussed in Chapter Three, people who try to lose weight too fast meet head-on with psychological and physiological barriers to self-control, which usually lead to relapse and weight regain. Therefore, it could be said that: *haste makes waist*. Take 6 to 12 months to change your eating style.

Advantages of Low-Fat Eating

One way to keep yourself motivated to stick to low-fat eating is that you can eat more food. If you enjoy eating, then low-fat eating is for you. Because low-fat food has fewer calories, you may find yourself eating much more quantity of food than you did when you were less careful. You can eat more food not only because the low-fat foods have fewer calories, but because body fat is related to the percentage fat in the diet.

For example, you can eat 8 ounces of broiled tuna, or 3.6 ounces of prime beef, or 2.5 ounces of Cheddar cheese, or half a small chicken pot pie, or 1.7 frankfurters, or 2 tablespoons of peanut butter. They all have about the same number of calories, but they are listed in increasing order of percent fat. If you were in a restaurant, and the waiter asked if you would prefer an 8-ounce fish steak or 2 tablespoons of peanut butter, which would you order?

Another advantage of eating low-fat foods is that you will be getting a better variety of nutrients in terms of vitamins and minerals from the greater quantity of foods you will be eating. When you start on your quest to become a low-fat eater, you can also thrill to the new recipes and even new foods you discover. You should never think of lower-fat eating in terms of hunger or deprivation. If you feel hungry and deprived, you are on a diet and will most likely relapse to old habits. The trick is gradually to reduce fat and at the same time to discover ways that you can satisfy yourself. The good news is that when a person reduces fat and exposure to high-fat foods, the desire to eat high-fat foods decreases.[3]

Visualization

One way to change the way you think and feel about high-fat foods is to recite the following poem. This poem is designed to allow you to visualize what is happening inside your body when you eat high-fat foods. It helps you to keep your focus on the truth about high-fat foods, and away from the enjoyable aspects of high-fat food ingestion. Some of our patients like this poem and put in on their refrigerators. Others hate it and don't use it. Decide for yourself whether it is motivational for you.

THE FAT POEM

Oh the joy of high-fat food!
Defends me from the outer world.
The comfort, the sensation, penetrating,
As I bite into a tasty morsel
Fat exploding upon my taste buds.
Oh that slimy, greasy fat
Bolting down my throat
Slithering into my stomach
And flowing in my veins.

This yellow gooey fat,
Building on artery walls,
Slowly accumulating there,
Clogging, blocking,
Cutting off blood to the brain,
Heart and other organs
Fostering debilitation.

The fat building under my skin
A yellow-greenish softening
Of my once proud body,
Now held in captivity
Of that high fat fate!
Oh the joy of high-fat food!

By G. Ken Goodrick and Phyllis Heyder-O'Donnell

Changing Your Food and Eating Environments

We do not live in a tropical rain forest. High-fat eating opportunities are thrust upon us everywhere. Can you drive to work without passing the exhaust vent of a fast-food restaurant? Can you go to the supermarket without seeing the mile-long aisle of chips? Most people can't. This is unfortunate because mere exposure to the sights and smells of high-fat foods can cause your body to increase insulin output, which lowers blood sugar level, which causes hunger to increase.[4] But this hunger is usually not the hunger related to food deprivation. This hunger is usually the instinctive hunger to store up calories as fat which was helpful thousands of years ago when food was scarce.

There are ways to change your food and eating environment to minimize the chances that you will be exposed to high-fat foods. Here are some methods to try:

- Keep all high-fat foods out of the house. If your spouse demands to have high-fat foods, let him/her buy and eat them elsewhere. If your children demand high-fat foods, let them know who is boss. (Consult with your pediatrician about when to reduce the fat in your children's eating. Some parents have overdone this and stunted their kids' growth.)

- Throw away all the deep-fat fryers you have.

- Avoid restaurants which feature high-fat foods (most do). Choose those which have healthful selections identified on the menu.

- Get T-shirts and lapel buttons made which say something like, *Low Fat is Where It's At*. This can help others know what you are trying to do, and help you resist high-fat eating.

- Eat with others who know about your goals.

- Join the Center for Science in the Public Interest. This is a consumer-advocacy group which focuses on nutritional problems of our food supply. You will get a newsletter which is educational and can be motivating. We have listed the Center in Appendix B.

Suzanne

Suzanne is a 29-year-old owner of a flower shop. Everyone in her family is overweight. She has been considerably overweight since early childhood. She realized that she was eating the wrong foods but couldn't control her temptation to eat high-fat treats. She had been on many diets but they were all short-lived. This is what she wrote after being in therapy for three months:

I guess I should tell you that I was sexually abused by a neighbor when I was 6 years old. Therapists have told me that this can really screw up self-esteem, and that I may be eating out of control because food represents the love that I feel I am unworthy of from others. Does that make sense? I am trying to learn to love myself with food that is less harmful for my weight problem.

In my family everything we ate was high in fat. My grandparents were farmers in Iowa and maybe they needed all those calories back in the 1920's. But our family kept on the tradition of heavy eating. We grew up on fried pork chops, potatoes with gravy and butter. All vegetables had butter on them.

121

Everyone smeared butter thick on bread. We never had a dinner without dessert. All dairy products were whole-fat, and we ate a lot of cheese. My grandparents and many family friends were dairy farmers. I remember my grandfather explaining to me the importance and desirability of lots of cream at the top of a milk bottle. We drank lemonade and soft drinks with sugar. I am getting sick just thinking of what we did to ourselves back then!

When I left home for college I knew that I was unacceptably fat. I did the diet stuff, and several programs taught me about nutrition and the evils of excess fat. But I found it impossible to stay away from my old favorites for very long. I would actually start a diet, then a few days into it I would go to the store and buy brownie mix and ice cream. I remember fixing it and eating it with pleasure but having negative thoughts about myself all the time I was doing it. It was like having a split personality.

I used to feel really deprived on diets. I guess you are supposed to feel deprived. Now I am learning that if you make yourself feel deprived, you are at war with yourself and you will end up the loser. Now I don't feel deprived by not eating high-fat foods, because my attitude toward high-fat foods is that they are damaging to health. So the true deprivation comes from eating high-fat treats.

I have learned to eat lower-fat substitutes which are enjoyable. I sometimes will have a giant green salad with vinegar, herbs, and sugar substitute. This is very filling and really low in fat. I think I have more energy when I stick to low-fat foods. I don't know if this is psychological or what. I do know that after a high-fat meal I felt like napping, which makes the situation worse. I do like to visualize less fat in my blood vessels. I like to read the "Fat Poem" to myself. I had it printed out in fancy letters on a computer, and framed it in my kitchen. My attitude toward high-fat foods has really become more negative, so that I am not tempted as much any more.

I have also called two friends from my group to help me get through three temptation crises. One time I was told over the phone to throw away two quarts of ice cream and to eat two apples. With someone telling me to do it, it seemed easy. After the crises, I felt really good.

I still have times when I splurge on high-fat foods, but much less often than I did before, and I don't get so upset about it.

Progress: Suzanne seems to be getting the message about high-fat foods. She is reporting a reduction of about 20 percent in fat grams on her food records. Her weight is coming down very slowly, but she seems to understand that a slow rate of weight loss is necessary in this program. She is also in a therapy group to deal with her history of abuse.

THE BOTTOM LINE:

- If you think of high-fat foods as *treats*, and feel deprived when you don't eat them, you may be haunted by thoughts of giving in to temptation. Eventually you will lose the battle.

- Gradually learn to think of foods with excessive fat content as less and less desirable, so that you automatically reject them. Many prepared foods have added fat to make them more tempting; don't be duped. Go for the lower-fat alternatives.

Awareness Exercises

1. Write down your memories of high-fat and high-sugar food treats which you enjoyed as a child. Did your mother make them especially for you?

_____

_____

_____

Nothing can replace the nurturing care of a good mother in childhood. But you can still feel nurtured with lower-fat food alternatives. Many of the foods which your mother gave you would be a mistake to eat too often today. But her love for you was not a mistake. Try to keep food and love separate.

2. Describe your feelings before, during, and after eating a large amount of high-fat food.

_____

_____

_____

Although such food may taste good, do you have negative feelings while you eat it? Can you really enjoy eating if you have guilt or shame hanging over your head? After overeating, don't you usually wish you hadn't? Focus on enjoyment of eating lower-fat foods.

3. Do you feel deprived if you don't eat high-fat, high-sugar foods? If you don't, then you should have little trouble switching to lower-fat, lower sugar alternatives. If you do, write down why you feel deprived.

    _____

    _____

    _____

    Try to realize that the real deprivation lies in what you are missing in terms of health and feelings of success when you eat high-fat, high-sugar foods. Try the latest foods made with fat substitutes.

4. Write down all the high-fat foods you enjoy now. Circle the ones you plan to eat only rarely after adopting the plan in this book.

    _____

    _____

    _____

    Reducing the fat in your eating doesn't mean you have to say goodbye forever to certain treats. You can still enjoy grandma's apple pie on holidays. A wedge of Aunt Emma's cheesecake is still a possibility. Your practice of eating lower-fat foods most of the time will allow a few deviations. And you can enjoy these deviations fully since they are eaten in the context of an otherwise prudent diet.

8

THE PLAN

First, make sure you're right. Then go ahead.[1]

Never, never, never, never, never, never, never give up.[2]

This chapter provides a concise, step-by-step plan for escaping your obese self and becoming your healthy self. The plan includes the three critical elements:

- Setting up a support system

- Establishing an exercise habit

- Establishing a low-fat eating habit

STEP 1
Read Chapters 1 - 7

Read Chapters One through Seven very carefully. Highlight in yellow the parts which are especially important to you. Make posters of motivational statements and hang them up throughout your house and place of work. Show this book to friends and explain your intent to follow through with this plan.

STEP 2
Complete the Self-Evaluation Form

Complete a Self-Evaluation Form in Appendix D so that you will have a record of how you were doing when starting this plan. Appendix D includes two extra Self Evaluation Forms so that you can evaluate yourself 6 and 12 months from now.

(Note: These self-evaluations are designed to help you evaluate your progress. They are not research-derived questionnaires, so don't compare scores amongst friends.)

STEP 3
See Your Physician

See your physician to make sure that this plan is medically safe for you. Show him or her this book. Your physician may want to perform some tests to determine if you have any hidden medical conditions which might limit your exercise program. Your eating plan may need to be modified if you have a medical problem requiring a special diet.

STEP 4
Get Social Support

Note: Some individuals have a real fear or dread of entering into the kind of group described in Chapter Five. Some are very shy, private people. It may be extremely difficult to discuss problems with others. Some may also be suffering from depression. These individuals may want to get therapy from a psychologist before entering a group. They should contact their local psychological association to find a clinical psychologist who can help.

Finding a group

Finding an existing group is easier than starting your own. Use the list below to aid in your search:

Overeaters Anonymous: Phone:—————————————

Meeting Places
and Times:—————————————————————

—————————————————————————

Psychologists/Therapists with ongoing groups:
Contact the International Association of Eating Disorders Professionals for member therapists near you. (See Appendix B).

—————————————————————————

—————————————————————————

Religious Organizations: Contact denominational headquarters for your area. You may be able to join or start a group at your place of worship.

_____

_____

_____

Psychiatric Hospitals: Some hospitals have therapy groups which may be similar to those recommended in this book. (They may want to sell you a treatment program. Get a second opinion before buying.)

_____

_____

_____

Dietitians: Contact your local Dietetic Association to see if registered dietitians are conducting weight management groups.

_____

_____

_____

When you find a group that looks promising, use the list below to check the quality of support offered.

- Helpful and friendly advice
- Encouragement
- Members share experiences
- Members share emotions
- Members are willing to confront me with the truth about myself
- I get feedback about myself
- Others try to boost my self-esteem
- Others make me feel I am normal
- Others are willing to help me through crises

Starting A Group

You may have one or more friends or associates who would like to work with you on escaping from your obese self. Here is an organizational policy statement which you can use as a guide for your group. Although this is written for women, it can be used for groups of men as well.

Organizational Policy

Name: The name of this group shall
be:_____

Membership: Open to all persons who are willing to work together to:

- Help each other increase self-acceptance.
- Help each other manage eating and exercise habits.

- Develop friendships to cope with rejection from the thin world.

Values: Members will strive to uphold these values:

- People should be accepted for who they are, not what their bodies look like.
- Health through exercise and low-fat eating is the goal, not any scale weight. Diets are dead.
- All behaviors should nurture. Self-nurturance should be in balance with nurturing others.
- In a crisis, it is better to reach out to others for help than to try to control oneself.
- Sharing life with others and being able to help are the keys to happiness.
- Concerns about weight and appearance should take up only a small portion of one's life.

Meetings: Meetings will be held weekly at a member's residence. Group meetings should have 8 or fewer members.

The format of meetings will be:

- Greetings and introductions of new members/visitors.
- Each member shares her successes and mistakes.
- Other members help analyze the reasons for mistakes and make suggestions.

- A discussion about self-esteem, social pressure to be thin, feelings of prejudice against the overweight or other mutually agreed-upon topics.
- Recitation of group's credo (based on Values). Prayer/giving thanks that can be shared with loving others.

Socializing: Members are encouraged to exercise together, eat low-fat meals together, and have low-fat parties.

Support: All members will give and get support as follows:

- All members' home and work phone numbers will be distributed on a support list.
- Members agree to be available by phone to help talk another member through a crisis. Visiting the member in crisis may also be needed.
- Members will call another member who fails to attend a group meeting without calling in advance with a reason. The absent member will be encouraged to keep attending.

Resignation: A member may resign from this group only if she appears before the group to state her reasons for leaving. Other members will encourage her to stay if they feel her leaving might be a step backward in her progress toward a healthy self. If the member fails to appear before the group to resign, other members will have at least three talks or phone calls with the leaving member encouraging her to rejoin. If she still desires to leave, a card will be sent after 3 months to let her know the group is still thinking of her.

These are the basics of a good support group. You may want to modify the policy to fit your particular needs. But don't get bogged down in rules. The group is for support, fun, and friendship.

Note: The support group is to be used as a resource to help you normalize your eating. Your peers can help you avoid overeating, and they can also help you avoid undereating. In the beginning of the Eating Plan, you may actually gain weight as a result of eating three meals a day. Weight loss will occur very gradually as your body adjusts to less fat in your meals. Use social support to help you avoid a return to dieting if your weight increases in the early part of your program.

STEP 5
Setting Your Goal Weight

Earlier in this book, we emphasized that weight and appearance shouldn't be your goals; that you shouldn't be motivated by vanity. Your goals should be to exercise and to eat less fat for health and energy. The weight you end up with when you eat and exercise prudently is your *optimal* weight in terms of mental and physical health.

However, we know there are some readers who will want to have a goal weight as a guide. Here are two ways to calculate goal weight (for females only):

Ideal weight =   100 lbs plus 5 lbs for each inch over 5 feet.

Example: If you are 5 feet 5 inches, your *Ideal* weight is about 125 pounds.

Remember: *Ideal weight* for most people is a fantasy which corresponds to the *socially acceptable* weight in a society obsessed with thinness.

Method 1:   Your goal weight can be calculated by a formula based on the experience of many patients who were able to maintain their weight losses.[3] This goal weight is equal to:

Ideal Weight

+

(Age + Number of years overweight) times 0.22

+

(Maximum weight ever) divided by 10

-

4.4

Example: A person who is 5 feet 5 inches tall, is 40 years old, has been overweight for 15 years, and had a maximum weight of 190 pounds, has a goal weight of:

125

+

(40 + 15) times 0.22, or 12.1

+

(190) divided by 10, or 19

-

4.4

= 152 lbs.

Method 2:   Another rule of thumb is that your goal
              weight should be no lower than the lowest
              weight you have been able to maintain for at
              least one year since you were 21 years old.[4]

Example: If you maintained a weight of 150 pounds
              for one year when you were 35, and you
              now weigh 190, your goal weight should be
              above 150 pounds.

There are two important things to consider about your goal weight:

- You may feel that your goal weight is still *fat*.
  Instead of rejecting this goal and trying to get
  thinner, reread Chapter Three and try to accept the
  fact that you may never be thin.
- It will take time to reach your goal. Accept the
  slow pace of healthful weight management.

Example: If you weighed 190 and your goal weight is
              150, it will take you 40 weeks to lose the
              weight at one pound per week. But since no
              one is perfect, plan on at least a full year.

STEP 6
Exercise Plan

The goal of this exercise plan is to help you gradually work up to four enjoyable 45-minute walks each week. Check with your physician before getting started. We recommend that you achieve this level of exercise before trying more strenuous forms of activity. This is a brief outline to get you started. Together with Chapter Six, it should be all you need. As you become more advanced, you may want to get the fitness books listed in Appendix B. You may also want to join a YWCA or YMCA where you can get expert exercise advice.

Here are some basic tips about walking so that you get started on the right foot.

What to Wear

Comfortable, loose clothing. Walking shoes, or at least shoes which feel comfortable. A watch to time yourself.

How to Walk

Keep your spine straight and hold your head high as you walk. Swing your arms. Don't worry about the length of your stride, just do what feels natural. Your heel should hit first, your foot rolls forward, and then you spring off your toes.

How Fast to Walk

Breathe deeply and walk at a comfortable rate. Walk at your normal speed, no matter how slow, for the first few weeks. Then, as you become accustomed to longer walks, try to walk as quickly as you can, slowing down if you feel uncomfortable or if your breathing is strained. You should always feel that walking is invigorating, never strenuous or burdensome.

There are ways to determine how fast you should walk. You can use these methods to self-regulate your speed.

- The *talk test*: you should be able to carry on a conversation while walking. If you can't, slow down.

- Your walk should be painless except perhaps for minor leg aches and soreness in the first few weeks. If you experience pain in your chest, jaw, or neck, STOP IMMEDIATELY and check with your physician.

- If, after walking, you feel excessively tired for an hour or longer, the walk was too strenuous. The next time, walk more slowly and not so far.

- Use your heart rate as a guide. A comfortable level is about 70% of your maximum. You cannot use heart rate as an absolute guide because many other factors such as emotion and environmental conditions can affect heart rate. A better guide is to use a range from between 60-80% of maximum. As your fitness level improves you can use your heart rate to regulate your exercise. When your heart rate is lower than usual it may be time to speed up.

TABLE 8.1[5]
Exercise Heart Rates
(As percent maximum capacity)

AGE YEARS	MEN 70% BEATS PER MINUTE	60-80% BEATS PER MINUTE
20	158	134-187
30	151	129-179
40	145	124-170
50	137	118-159
60	130	113-151
70	123	108-142

AGE YEARS	WOMEN 70% BEATS PER MINUTE	60-80% BEATS PER MINUTE
20	161	132-181
30	154	128-174
40	148	124-166
50	140	118-155
60	133	114-148
70	126	110-141

When to Walk

Try to pick a walking time which is least likely to interfere with your normal schedule. Some people like to walk at dawn before breakfast, others after dinner. There are some people who normally hate to get up early who have found that an early morning walk gives them more energy to start their day. Others, who feel exhausted after a day of taking care of children or working in an office, find that an evening walk refreshes them both physically and mentally.

Never walk in the heat of a summer's day. Walk where it is safe: in shopping malls, or in parks where there are other exercisers present.

Options

You can try exercising at home on a treadmill, stepping machine, or stationary bicycle. Just be sure to follow the exercise intensity rules of self-regulation. An advantage of home exercise is that you can watch television or even read a book while exercising. You can also control the weather indoors.

Frequency and Duration of Walks

If you are not accustomed to exercise walking, start with a 5-minute walk. If you think this is too easy, try 10 minutes the next time. After a few days you should discover how long you can walk without feeling too tired afterward. A good general rule is to add five minutes to each walk each week. For example:

Week 1 : 4 walks, 10 minutes each
Week 2 : 4 walks, 15 minutes each
Week 3 : 4 walks, 20 minutes each

Keep adding five minutes until you are doing four 45-minute walks each week. But always go by how you feel. Let your body and not your mind decide how much exercise to do. Don't overdo it.

Keeping Track of Your Progress

In order for you to monitor your exercise habit development, keep an exercise diary on a calendar or in your appointment book. This way you can look back over time to see how consistently you have been exercising. Remember that habit development may be slow. It may take you 6 to 12 months to get to the point where you are a regular exerciser. Don't rush yourself. A Daily Self-Monitoring form is included in the next section which has a place to record exercise as well as foods eaten.

STEP 7
The Eating Plan

The goals of the eating plan are:

- to gradually reduce the fat in the diet down to about 30 percent of calories;
- to eat three meals a day, with two between-meal snacks if needed;
- to eat in a balanced way from all the food groups.

Reducing Fat in the Diet

There are two ways to achieve this goal: the easy way, and the mathematical way.

The easy way: Eat only low-fat foods consisting of:

- whole grains
- fruits, beans, and vegetables (but not nuts, seeds, or avocados)
- low-fat dairy products
- trimmed lean meats, poultry and fish

A general rule to follow is: avoid foods which are prepared with fat (fried) or which have fat as an added ingredient (e.g., gravy, croissants).

If you limit yourself to only low-fat foods, the percentage of calories from fat will remain low no matter how much you eat. However, it is possible to gain weight eating only low-fat foods if the total calories are high. Therefore, be careful to follow the recommended number of servings per day shown in the Recommended Daily Eating Plan. There is a colorful poster called *The New American Eating Guide* (Appendix B) which categorizes foods according to whether they are low, medium, or high in fat. We recommend that this poster decorate a wall of your kitchen so that you can easily select low-fat foods.

The mathematical way to reduce fat in the diet: Calculate your daily fat gram intake by keeping a food diary (Daily Record). Appendix E is a partial list of foods showing how many grams of fat are in normal servings. A more complete list can be found in a handy little book called *The fat counter and the 22-gram solution* (See Appendix B).

Record everything you eat on the Daily Record. Add up the fat grams you have eaten each day for a week. Divide by seven to get your daily average fat gram intake.

The above calculations are based on where you are now. In order to find your fat grams per day goal, you will need to recalculate based on your goal weight. Here is the formula:

Goal weight times 14 (13 if you aren't exercising, 15 if you exercise a lot) minus ten times (Age - 25) equals calories per day at your goal weight.

Figure this for yourself:

Goal weight_____ times 14 = _____ (A)

Age Factor is 10 times (age-25) = _____ (B)

Subtract (B) from (A) = _____
This is your goal calories per day

Example: Jane's goal weight is 150, times 14 equals 2100 calories per day, minus her age factor,[10 times (40-25), or 150], equals 1950 calories per day.

Now, multiply your goal calories per day by 30 percent to get fat calories per day:
Goal calories per day _____ times 0.30 = _____
This is your fat calories per day.

Divide fat calories per day by 9 to get fat grams per day.

Fat calories per day _____ divided by 9 = _____

This is your goal fat grams per day.

Note: If your current daily fat gram intake is equal to or less than your goal fat grams per day, and you are eating a reasonable amount and variety of foods, you are already eating prudently. Your emphasis should be on exercise.

Example: Jane's goal fat calories per day is 1950 times 0.30 = 585 calories from fat per day.

Divide 585 by 9 to get 65 grams of fat per day.

Note: Remember that the above formulas are estimations; the numbers you calculate for yourself may not be precise. But you should be able to get a general idea of how your current fat gram consumption compares with your goal.

In order to change your eating habits gradually, reduce the fat in your eating slowly so that you achieve your fat grams goal over a period of 6 to 12 months.

The overall goal is to reduce fat grams from where you are now to your goal fat grams per day. This should be done slowly, as you select and prepare foods which are lower in fat.

What to Eat

As you record fat grams, you should quickly learn which foods are higher in fat. About 12 months from now, you should be avoiding butter, margarine, gravy, salad dressing that is not non-fat, and other food products which sneak excess fat into their recipes. You should also avoid sugary foods; for a sweet taste, stick to fruit.

As for what foods to eat, the following guidelines are offered. You need not eat exactly the recommended portions every day, but there should be a good representation of the food groups over each week.

THE RECOMMENDED DAILY EATING PLAN[6]

FOOD GROUP	SERVINGS/DAY
Vegetables	3-5 servings
Fruits	2-4 servings
Breads, cereals, rice, and pasta	6-11 servings
Milk, yogurt, and cheese	2-3 servings
Meats, poultry, fish, dry beans and peas, and eggs	2-3 servings

Servings are defined according to the food group. For vegetables count as one serving 1 cup of raw leafy greens, ½cup of other kinds. One serving of fruits is one medium apple, orange, or banana; ½ cup of small or diced fruit; ¾ cup of juice. One serving from the bread category is 1 slice of bread; ½ bun, bagel, or english muffin; 1 ounce of dry ready-to-eat cereal; ½ cup of cooked cereal, rice, or pasta. For a serving of milk products have 1 cup of milk or yogurt or about 1½ ounces of cheese. You should consume a total of about 6 ounces of meat daily to equal 2-3 servings.

As you get into the habit of eating low-fat, low-sugar foods, and eating three meals a day, your compulsion to overeat or binge will diminish. Your cravings for inappropriate foods will become less frequent. You will begin to eat *normally*.

What to Drink

Many overweight persons tend to drink less water than they need for good health, possibly because they do not want to add water weight, or because drinking makes them feel over-full. The irony is that if you don't drink enough water, the body may try to retain fluids so that your tissues will maintain a proper fluid/electrolyte balance. You may have less water retention if you drink more water. We recommend 8 to 12 glasses a day.

Record Keeping

To keep track of what you are eating, and to learn about the fat content of foods, it is essential that you keep a fat-gram log for at least two months. You can use the Daily Eating and Exercise Record for Beginners to keep track of what you have eaten and how you have exercised every day. Make copies of this form for your personal use, or make up your own form. After you learn which foods have the highest and lowest fat, use the Daily Eating and Exercise Record for Advanced Users. You should keep records until you feel you are in good control of eating and exercise. This may take up to a year. Always return to record keeping when you feel you are losing control. Along with social support, it can be a powerful tool to help you get back on track.

_____, 19___ .

FOOD	AMOUNT	FAT GRAMS
	TOTAL FAT GRAMS	
FLUID (8oz.)	1 2 3 4 5 6 7 8 9 10	
EXERCISE: WHAT_____	DURATION: _____	HOW I FELT: _____

Daily Eating and Exercise Record for Beginners

(Record "L" for low-fat, "H" for high-fat for each serving)

Vegetables ☐☐☐☐☐

Fruits ☐☐☐☐

Breads, cereals, ☐☐☐☐☐☐☐☐☐☐
rice, & pasta

Milk, yogurt, & ☐☐☐
cheese

Meats, poultry, fish, ☐☐☐
dry beans and peas, & eggs

Fluid (8 oz. servings) 1 2 3 4 5 6 7 8

Exercise: What:_____ Duration:_____

Daily Eating and Exercise Record for Advanced Users

Also put up a wall calendar in your home. Put an *L* on each day you ate only low-fat foods. Put an *E* on each day you exercised. At the end of the month count the L and E days. Over a year, you will see the number of E and L days per month increasing. This calendar recording is designed to remind you that changes take time, and there will be times when you revert back to your old ways. But if you stick to the plan, you will eventually arrive at your destination: Happier, healthier, and a little thinner.

APPENDIX A

GETTING PROFESSIONAL HELP[1]

This appendix is designed to help you evaluate weight clinics in order to find one which can best help you follow the principles outlined in this book.

Your Special Psychological Needs

Before you seek help with weight management, think about your emotional needs. Some overweight persons, either due to unfortunate childhood circumstances such as abuse or neglect, or due to their poor self-image, become socially isolated as adults. Their only friends may be fellow overweight persons who share their sorrows more than they try to lift each other up. Some overweight persons have higher than normal levels of anxiety or depression, which may go hand-in-hand with binge eating. Some seek weight control as a solution to depression and social isolation.

If improved emotions is one of your weight-loss goals, find a clinic which can arrange psychological counseling. This counseling can help you be realistic about how your life might change when you achieve a reasonable amount of weight loss. Most persons find that weight loss does not solve their serious psychological or relationship problems. Worse, after weight loss, they are less able to use overweight as an excuse for their problems, and they have to face the possibility that the problems are more complex than weight loss.

Looking at Programs

Treatment focus

When you select a weight management clinic, look for one which will help you achieve your maximum state of physical and mental health. For overweight persons, this will require an emphasis on at least three treatment components: 1) reduction of excess fat in your eating habits, down to about 30 percent of total calories; 2) increase in physical activity such as walking to about four hours per week; and 3) counseling to help you accept your body appearance at the weight you achieve.

Long-term approach

Any program you select should be designed for a lifetime approach. Weight management is not a one-shot attempt to lose weight. It is a life-long adoption of healthful eating and physical activity habits. A program should offer follow-up classes for as long as you want to attend them. The program should recommend a rate of weight loss of no more than 1 pound per week. The health professionals you hire should help you accept the slow pace of successful weight management, and do what they can to keep you motivated.

Ethics and professionalism

A clinic should be staffed with licensed physicians, registered dietitians, and licensed counselors so that you will get treatment offered by professionals who are ethically bound to provide you with the most effective methods known. They can give you a thorough medical, nutritional, and psychological assessment so that your treatment program will be tailored to your specific needs, in order to deal with the complex nature of obesity.

A licensed health professional should also want to discuss with you before treatment begins exactly what your individual problems are, what the treatment will involve, what the dangers and drawbacks might be, and what level of success you can expect to achieve. All costs should be revealed before you spend a penny.

There are many programs which operate with questionable ethics or which practice fraud; the weight-loss industry is not very well regulated by government agencies, although this may soon happen. You need to proceed with caution if a program:

- Promises quick or easy weight loss.

- Relies on testimonials from their most successful clients.

- Refrains from giving you detailed program information or prices unless you visit their clinic first.

- Uses methods which are not reported in scientific journals as helpful (such as body wrapping, injections, all-fruit diets, herbs, etc.).

Program Quiz

Use this quiz as a guide to evaluate any program you are thinking about joining. If you are going to pay your own money to get help with weight management, you have a right to make sure the program meets the highest standards. Take this quiz to the clinic you are investigating and go over each item carefully. Mark each item as either *P* for pass or *F* for fail. Don't talk to a salesperson; get your questions answered by a health professional.

EVALUATING WEIGHT MANAGEMENT CLINICS QUIZ

1. Does the weight management clinic provide for medical and psychological screening?   P F
2. Does the clinic help you with out-of-control binge eating?   P F
3. Is an assessment of your body composition (percent body fat) done?   P F
4. Is counseling provided by persons licensed to practice?   P F
5. Is nutrition taught by registered dietitians (RD)?   P F
6. Is exercise instructed by certified persons (e.g., by the American College of Sports Medicine?)   P F
7. Is medical supervision done by licensed physicians who are present at the clinic for more than quick visits?   P F

8.   Do you get a written estimate of the total costs to you and the schedule of treatment and follow-up classes recommended for you?   P F

9.   Do you get a written informed consent form which states the benefits and risks to you, how much you can expect to lose, what the drop-out rate is for the clinic's clients, and what the success rate is for this clinic?   P F

10. Is the goal weight recommended for you based on family history of obesity, your body composition and weight-loss history, not on charts?   P F

11. Is the emphasis in treatment on achieving optimal physical and mental health?   P F

12. Is the rate of weight loss one pound per week or less (unless medically-supervised very-low-calorie-diet)?   P F

13. Does the program encourage you to get the recommended dietary allowance (RDA) of vitamins and minerals, no less and not much more?   P F

14. Does the medical exam include an evaluation for exercise?   P F

15. Does the exercise program goal recommend a gradual increase to about 4 hours of physical activity each week, based on how much you can do and still feel comfortable and energetic?   P F

16. Does the psychological component teach behavior modification techniques for changing eating and physical activity patterns, with a strong emphasis on social support in groups?   P F

17. Does the psychological component emphasize the cultural pressures to be thin, how self-esteem is often linked with body image, and how to develop a better self-image regardless of appearance?   P F

18. Does the clinic rely on appetite suppressant medications?   P F

19. Does the clinic provide a maintenance follow-up program which you can attend indefinitely for continuing support?   P F

20. Does the clinic give you copies of the scientific research published by others in scientific journals showing the results of the methods used?   P F

21. If you pay in advance for maintenance classes, does the contract specify that your money will be refunded to a charity rather than kept by the clinic if you decide to drop out?   P F

22. Can the clinic address your special ethnic needs?   P F

ANSWERS TO PROGRAM QUIZ

1. Careful screening is needed to tailor a program to your individual case. For example, you may already be exercising but need help with reducing fat in your diet.

2. If your dietary behavior involves binge eating, and you feel that you really are unable to control your intake of food, the program should provide counseling to help you understand how binge eating habits get started, and how to reduce out-of-control overeating. This will require group therapy to provide the kind of social support described in Chapter Five. The counseling should include a psychological evaluation with interviews and/or tests to determine your level of depression, anxiety, relationship problems, and symptoms of eating disorders such as binges, purges, and excessive feelings of shame over being unable to control eating. If you feel extremely uncomfortable in groups, you may want to try individual counseling first. One of the goals of this counseling would be to try to make you feel more at ease with others, since the ability to give and receive social support is a key to success and emotional well-being in general.

3. The amount of fat you have may determine your realistic goal weight. If you have lots of muscle, you can't expect to lose a lot of muscle healthfully in order to lose weight. Also, if you have a very high percentage of body fat, this may indicate that you have an overabundance of fat cells. These cells have a lower limit in size which may restrict how much you can reduce in body size.

4. Don't turn your personal and weight management problems over to someone who hasn't the proper training and experience. Licensed counselors will at a minimum have masters degrees and supervised experience, and are required to adhere to a professional code of ethics which inhibits them from exploiting you or from using untested methods.

5. There have been so many weird ideas about weight management and nutrition that it can really pay to make sure that your nutrition consultant is a registered dietitian who has training in the scientifically valid approaches to sound nutrition and sensible weight control.

6. Certified exercise instructors are required to keep your physical activity program safe.

7. Some programs advertise medical supervision by licensed physicians, but the M.D. only spends a few minutes a week at the clinic checking records.

8. Get everything in writing before you spend money. You are entering into a business contract. Read the fine print.

9. The risks and benefits of the program, the predicted realistic weight outcome for you, and the success rate for the clinic should be made known before you pay.

10. Your goal weight probably should be about halfway between what you weigh now and your ideal weight from the charts. (See Chapter Eight).

11. The way to optimal mental and physical health for the overweight person involves increasing physical activity, reducing fat in the diet, and accepting the weight you achieve after you have adopted healthful lifestyle changes. In other words, as discussed in Chapter Four, the clinic should not appeal to your vanity, but strive to help you be healthier and more self-accepting.

12. Faster rates of loss may cause you to relapse or become ill.

13. There is no evidence that excessive supplementation of any vitamins or minerals will have a beneficial effect on weight loss or maintenance.

14. A physician should go through a checklist to make sure you are not at a high level of risk to suffer injuries to legs or feet, or to damage your heart.

15. The physical activity program should be gradual, based on how you respond to exercise, so that physical pain can be minimized, and maximum enjoyment obtained from exercise.

16. Behavior modification is the best way to learn to change your eating and physical activity habits. Social support should be used to help you through crises.

17. The cultural pressures to be thin are thought to be among the primary causes of eating disorders. Some overweight persons may have low self-esteem because of their perceived inability to control weight, and because of the prejudices against the obese which they experience. Dealing with these feelings and prejudices should be an important part of any program.

18. Appetite suppressants are only effective for relatively short periods of time, and may cause harmful physical and psychological side effects if used for longer periods.

19. Long-term support through counseling or groups seems to be needed for many to help them maintain new eating and physical activity habits.

20. There have been so many fraudulent weight-loss treatments that you can't be too careful.

21. The incentive for both you and the clinic should be to keep you in the program.

22. The cultural and family rules you live with may influence your eating and exercise. If your spouse wants you to stay overweight, or if all your friends are overweight and not concerned about reducing, your weight management clinic should be able to provide some help in how to deal with resistance from others. If your cultural heritage requires you to prepare high-fat ethnic foods, your clinic's dietitian will be able to work with you to develop similar, lower-fat recipes which should help to satisfy your family.

APPENDIX B

RESOURCES

Magazines /Newsletters

BBW (Big Beautiful Woman)
P.O.B. 16958
North Hollywood, CA 91615-9964
Tel: (800) 245-4229

Radiance
P.O.B. 31703
Oakland, CA 94604
Tel: (415) 482-0680

These two magazines feature stories on fashion, self-esteem, relationships, and other topics of interest to large women.

Obesity & Health
Healthy Living Institute
Route 2, Box 905
Hettinger, ND 58639
Tel: (701) 567-2845

Weight Control Digest
1555 W. Mockingbird Lane, Suite 205
Dallas, TX 75235
Tel: (800) 736-7323

These two newsletters cover the latest research on obesity and tips from the experts.

Eating, Recipes, Nutrition

Brody, J. (1985). *Good food book: eating the high-carbohydrate way.* New York: Norton.

Brody, J. (1987). *Jane Brody's nutrition book.* New York: Bantam.

Callaway, C.W. (1990). *The Callaway diet: Successful permanent weight control for starvers, stuffers and skippers.* New York: Bantam Books.

Colorado Dietetic Association. (1989). *Simply Colorado: Nutritious recipes for busy people.* Littleton, Colorado: Author. 6939 South Benis Street.

Cooking Light: The Magazine of Food and Fitness.
P.O.Box 830549
Birmingham, AL 35282-9810
Tel: (800) 999-1750

DeBakey, M.E. *et al.* (1994). *The living heart brand name shoppers' guide.* New York: Mastermedia Ltd.

DeBakey, M.E. *et al.* (1986). *The living heart diet.* New York: Simon & Schuster.

Dwyer, J. & St. Jeor, S.(due 1992). *The optimal diet.* Dallas, TX: American Health Publishing Co.

Kaiser Permanente. (1991). *Health counts: A fat and calorie guide.* New York: John Wiley & Sons, Inc.

Lowfat Lifeline
52 Condolea Court
Lake Oswego, OR 97035
Tel: (503) 636-1559

This is a catalogue of products and books to help you follow a low-fat eating style.

Netzer, C.T. (1987). *The fat counter and the 22-gram solution.* New York: Dell.

Ponchitera, B.J. (1991). *Quick & Healthy: Recipes and ideas.* The Dalles, Oregon: Author. 1519 Hermits Way.

Scanlon, D. (1991). *Diets that work. For weight control or medical needs.* Los Angeles: Contemporary Books.

Spear, R. (1991). *Low fat and loving it: How to lower your fat intake and still eat the foods you love. 200 delicious recipes.* New York: Warner Books.

Warshaw, H.S. (1990). *The restaurant companion. A guide to healthier eating out.* Chicago, IL: Surrey Books.

Weight Management Computer

DietMate
PICS
12007 Sunridge Valley, Suite 480
Reston, VA 22091
Tel: (800) 343-8628

CALTRAC
20100 Hamilton
Torrance, CA
90502
Tel: (310) 715-8036

Movie

Jaglom, H. (Director) (1991). *Eating.*

Organizations

Calorie Control Council (CCC)
Suite 500-G
5775 Peachtree-Dunwoody Road
Atlanta, GA 30342
Tel: (404) 252-3663

CCC publishes the latest information on low-calorie products and sensible eating plans.

Center for Science in the Public Interest (CSPI)
1875 Connecticut Ave. N.W. Suite 300
Washington, D.C. 20009-5728
Tel: (202) 667-7483

CSPI publishes Nutrition Action Healthletter, a newsletter helpful for those trying to eat more healthfully. They also have a great poster, New American Eating Guide, which is useful in making low-fat food choices.

Largely Positive
P.O.B. 17223
Glendale, WI 53217

National Association for the Advancement of Fat
Acceptance (NAAFA)
P.O.Box 188620
Sacramento, CA 95818
Tel: (916) 443-0303

The previous two groups focus on helping enhance self-esteem among large people.

Overeaters Anonymous
World Service Office
P.O.B. 92870
Los Angeles, CA 90009
Tel: (213) 542-8363

An excellent organization for compulsive overeaters.

Books about Women and Weight

Bass, E., & Davis, L. (1988). *The courage to heal: A guide for women survivors of child sexual abuse.* New York: Harper and Row.

Women who were abused as children have an increased risk of becoming obese.

Bennett, W. & Gurin, J. (1982). *The dieter's dilemma: Eating less and weighing more.* New York: Basic Books.

Gürze Books (Mail order catalog)
P.O.B. 2238
Carlsbad, CA 92008-9883
Tel: (619) 434-7533

Books, tapes, and videos on eating disorders and other areas of interest to an individual's psychological growth.

Harrison, M., & Stewart-Roache, C. (1989). *AttrACTIVE woman: A physical fitness approach to emotional and spiritual well-being.* Park Ridge,IL: Parkside Publishing.
205 West Touhy Ave.
Park Ridge, IL 60068
Tel: (800) 221-6364

Kano, S. (1989). *Making peace with food: Freeing yourself from the diet/weight obsession* (Rev. Ed.). New York: Harper & Row.

Orbach, S. (1982). *Fat is a feminist issue.* New York: Berkeley Books.

Exercise Resources

Blair, S.N. (1991). *Living with exercise: Improving your health through moderate physical activity.* Dallas,TX: American Health Publishing.(Tel: 800-736-7323)

Books On Tape, Inc.
P.O. Box 7900
Newport Beach, CA 92658
Tel: (800) 626-3333

Recorded books for use while walking, jogging, or on stationary exercise bikes.

Hooked on Walking
Movin' In Sound, Inc.
P.O. Box 885
Cypress, TX 77429

Music for beginners and advanced. Keeps you in an aerobic pace.

Jackson, A.S., & Ross, R.M. (1992). *Understanding exercise for health and fitness.* Houston, TX: CSI Software, Inc.

Jive Bunny and the Master Mixers: The Album
Atco Records
75 Rockefeller Plaza
New York, NY 10019

JPF's favorite tape for jogging.

Lyons, P., & Burgard, D. (1990). *Great shape: the first fitness guide for large women.* Palo Alto, CA: Bull Publishing.

Recorded Books, Inc.
270 Skipjack Rd.
Prince Frederick, MD 20678
Tel: (800) 638-1304

Recorded books for use while walking, jogging, or on stationary exercise bikes.

Walking Magazine
Raben Publishing
711 Boylston Street
Boston, MA 02116
Tel: (617) 236-1885

Depression, Happiness, and Stress Books

Burns, D. (1980). *Feeling good*. New York: Morrow.

A great book for understanding and alleviating depression.

Charlesworth, E., & Nathan, R. (1982). *Stress management: A comprehensive guide to wellness*. New York: Ballantine.

A handbook everyone should use.

Fordyce, M.W. (due 1992). *The psychology of happiness: Its nature and attainment*. Ft. Myers, Fl: Cypress Lake Media.

For other materials on happiness, write to:
Professor Michael Fordyce, Edison Community College, Ft. Myers, Fl 33906.

Behavior Modification for Weight Management

Brownell, K.D. (1990). *The LEARN program for weight control*. Dallas, TX: The LEARN Education Center.
1555 Mockingbird Lane, Suite 203
Dallas, TX 75235
Tel: (800) 736-7323

Therapists

International Association of Eating Disorders Professionals
(IAEDP).
123 NW 13th Street, Suite 206
Boca Raton, FL 33432
Tel: (407) 338-6494

This organization can refer you to a therapist in your area.

APPENDIX C

REFERENCES

Preface

1. Foreyt, J.P., Goodrick,G.K., & Gotto, A.M. (1982). Evaluating commercial weight loss clinics. *Archives of Internal Medicine*, *142*, 682-683.

2. Goodrick, G.K., & Foreyt, J.P. (1991). Why treatments for obesity don't last. *Journal of the American Dietetic Association*, *91*, 1243-1247.

3. Lustig, A. (1991). Weight loss programs: Failing to meet ethical standards? *Journal of the American Dietetic Association*, *91*, 1252-1254.

4. Begley, C.E. (1991). Government should strengthen regulation in the weight loss industry. *Journal of the American Dietetic Association*, *91*, 1255-1257.

5. Wooley, S.C., & Garner, D.M. (1991). Obesity treatment: The high cost of false hope. *Journal of the American Dietetic Association*, *91*, 1248-1251.

6. Garner, D.M., & Wooley, S.C. (1991). Confronting the failure of behavioral and dietary treatments for obesity. *Clinical Psychology Review, 11*, 729-780.

Chapter One

1. Attributed to Robert B. Lockard, as described in Willems, E.P.(1974). Go ye into all the world and modify behavior: An ecologist's view. In S. Martin and B.J. Williams, (Eds.), *The child in his environment: Applications of behavioral ecology*. Houston, TX: Authors.

Chapter Two

1. Centers for Disease Control. (1989). Prevalence of overweight: Behavioral risk factor surveillance system, 1987. *Morbidity and Mortality Weekly Report*, *38*, 421-423.

2. National Center for Health Statistics. (1987). *Anthropometric reference data and prevalence of overweight. United States 1976-1980*. Hyattsville, Maryland: U.S. Department of Health and Human Services, Public Health Service, DHHS publication no. (PHS) 87-1688.

3. Van Itallie, T.B. (1985). Health implications of overweight and obesity in the United States. *Annals of Internal Medicine*, *103*, 983-988.

4. Bouchard, C., Tremblay A., Despres, J.P., Nadeau, A., Lupien, R.J., Theriault, G., Dussalt, J., Moorjani, S., Pinault, S., & Fournier, G. (1990). The response to long-term overfeeding in identical twins. *New England Journal of Medicine*, *322*, 1477-1482.

5. Stunkard, A.J., Foch, T.T., & Hrubec, Z. (1986). A twin study of human obesity. *Journal of the American Medical Association, 256,* 51-54.

6. Stunkard, A.J., Harris, J.R., Pedersen, N.L., & McClearn, G.E. (1990). The body mass index of twins who have been reared apart. *New England Journal of Medicine, 322,* 1483-1487.

7. Stunkard, A.J., Sorensen, T.I.A., Hanis, C., Teasdale, T.W., Chakraborty, R., Schull, W.J., & Schulsinger, F. (1986). An adoption study of human obesity. *New England Journal of Medicine, 314,* 193-198.

8. Ravussin, E., Lillioja, S., Knowler, W.C., Christin, L., Freymond, D., Abbott, W.G.H., Boyce, V., Howard, B.V., & Bogardus, C. (1988). Reduced rate of energy expenditure as a risk factor for body-weight gain. *New England Journal of Medicine, 318,* 467-472.

9. Roberts, S.B., Savage, J., Coward, W.A., Chew, B., & Lucas, A. (1988). Energy expenditure and intake in infants born to lean and overweight mothers. *New England Journal of Medicine, 318,* 461-466.

10. Brownell, K.D., Greenwood, M.R.C., Stellar, E., & Shrager, E.E. (1986). The effects of repeated cycles of weight loss and regain in rats. *Physiology and Behavior, 38,* 459-464.

Chapter Three

1. Bennett,W. & Gurin, J. (1982) *The dieter's dilemma*. New York: Basic Books.

2. Rodin, J., Radke-Sharpe, N., Rebuffe-Scrive,M., & Greenwood, M.R.C. (1990). Weight cycling and fat distribution. *International Journal of Obesity*, *14*, 303-310.

3. Lissner, L., Odell, P.M., D'Agostino,R.B., et al. (1991). Variability of body weight and health outcomes in the Framingham population. *New England Journal of Medicine*, *324*, 1839-44.

4. Polivy, J., & Herman, C.P. (1985). Dieting and binging: A causal analysis. *American Psychologist*, *40*, 193-201.

5. Sjoberg,L., & Persson,L. (1977). A study of attempts by obese persons to regulate eating. *Goteborg Psychological Reports*, *7*, No. 12.

6. Wooley, S.C., & Garner, D.M. (1991). Obesity treatment: The high cost of false hope. *Journal of the American Dietetic Association*, *91*, 1248-1251.

7. Schlundt, D.G., Sbrocco, T., & Bell, C. (1989). Identification of high-risk situations in a behavioral weight-loss program: Application of the relapse prevention model. *International Journal of Obesity*, *13*, 223-234.

8. Schlundt, D.G., Hill, J.O., Sbrocco, T., Pope-Cordle, J., & Kasser,T. (1990). Obesity: A biogenetic or biobehavioral problem. *International Journal of Obesity, 14,* 815-828.

9. American Psychiatric Association (1987). *Diagnostic and statistical manual of mental disorders.* 3rd ed., rev. Washington,D.C.: American Psychiatric Press.

10. Gormally, J., Black, S., Daston, S., & Rardin, D. (1982). The assessment of binge eating severity among obese persons. *Addictive Behaviors, 7,* 47-55.

11. Loro, A.D., & Orleans, C.S. (1981). Binge eating in obesity: Preliminary findings and guidelines for behavioral analysis and treatment. *Addictive Behaviors, 6,* 155-166.

12. Wilson, G.T. (1991). The addiction model of eating disorders: A critical analysis. *Advances in Behavior Research and Therapy, 13,* 27-72.

13. Miller, W. C. (1991). Diet composition, energy intake, and nutritional status in relation to obesity in men and women. *Medicine and Science in Sports and Exercise, 23,* 280-284.

14. Tremblay, A., Lavallee, N., Almeras, N., Allard, L., Despres, J-P., & Bouchard, C. (1991). Nutritional determinants of the increase in energy intake associated with a high-fat diet. *American Journal of Clinical Nutrition, 53,* 1134-1137.

15.   Kendall, A., Levitsky, D.A., Strupp, B.J., & Lissner, L. (1991). Weight loss on a low-fat diet: Consequence of the imprecision of the control of food intake in humans. *AMerican Journal of Clinical Nutrition, 53*, 1124-1129.

Chapter Four

1.   From Office of Student Affairs, Smith College, Northampton, MA.

2.   Adapted from Ecclesiastes. (1986). *The Bible*. New International Version.

3.   Fernando, aka Billy Crystal.

4.   Brumberg, J.J. (1988). *Fasting girls: The emergence of anorexia nervosa as a modern disease.* Cambridge, Ma: Harvard University Press.

5.   Foreyt, J.P. & Goodrick, G.K. (1982). Gender and obesity. In I.Al-Issa (Ed.), *Gender and psychopathology*. New York: Academic Press.

6.   Rozin, P., & Fallon, A. (1988). Body image, attitudes to weight, and misperceptions of figure preferences of the opposite sex: A comparison of men and women in two generations. *Journal of Abnormal Psychology, 97*, 342-245.

7.   Harris, L. (1987). *Inside America*. New York: Vintage Books.

8.   Glassner, B. (1988). *Bodies: Why we look the way we do and how we feel about it.* New York: Putnam.

9.   Orbach, S. (1982). *Fat is a feminist issue.* New York: Berkeley Books.

10.   Ciliska, D. (1990). *Beyond dieting: Psychoeducational interventions for chronically obese women.* New York: Brunner/Mazel.

Chapter Five

1.   Adapted from John Donne.

2.   Adapted from Ecclesiastes. (1986). *The Bible.* New International Version.

3.   McCarthy, M. (1990). The thin ideal, depression and eating disorders in women. *Behaviour Research and Therapy, 28,* 205-215.

4.   Kuskowska-Wolk, A., & Rossner, S. (1990) Social isolation and obesity. *International Journal of Obesity, 14* (Suppl 2), 55 (Abstract).

5.   Miller, C.T., Rothblum, E.D., Barbour, L., Brand, P.A., & Felicio, D. (1990). Social interactions of obese and non-obese women. *Journal of Personality, 58,* 365-380.

6.   Kayman, S., Bruvold, W., & Stern, J.S. (1990). Maintenance and relapse after weight loss in women: Behavioral aspects. *American Journal of Clinical Nutrition, 52,* 800-807.

7.   Foreyt, J.P., & Goodrick, G.K. (1991). Factors common to successful treatment for the obese patient. *Medicine and Science in Sports and Exercise, 23,* 292-297.

8.   Levy, L.H. (1979). Processes and activities in groups. In M.A. Lieberman, L.D. Borman & Associates (Eds.), *Self-help groups for coping with crisis.* San Francisco, CA: Jossey-Bass.

9.   Sobal, J. (1984). Group dieting, the stigma of obesity, and overweight adolescents: Contributions of Natalie Allon to the sociology of obesity. *Marriage and Family Review, 7,* 9-20.

10.   Overeaters Anonymous. (1988). *A survey of Overeaters Anonymous groups and membership in North America.* Torrance, CA: Author.

11.   Callaway, C.W. (1990). *The Callaway diet: Successful permanent weight control for starvers, stuffers, and skippers.* New York: Bantam Books.

Chapter Six

1.   National Geographic television special.

2. Griest, J.H., Eischens, R.R., Klein, M.H., & Faris, J.W. (1979). Antidepressant running. *Psychiatric Annals, 9*, 134-140.

3. Reed, D.R., Contreras, R.J., Maggio, C., Greenwood, M.R., & Rodin, J. (1988). Weight cycling in female rats increases dietary fat selection and adiposity. *Physiology and Behavior, 42*, 389-395.

4. Gerardo-Gettens, T., Miller, G.D., Horwitz, B.A., McDonald, R.B., Brownell, K.D., Greenwood, M.R., Rodin, J., & Stern, J.S. (1991). Exercise decreases fat selection in female rats during weight cycling. *American Journal of Physiology, 260*, R518-524.

Chapter Seven

1. Daniel (1986). *The Bible*. New International Version.

2. Danguir, J. (1987). Cafeteria diet promotes sleep in rats. *Appetite*, 8, 40-53.

3. Mattes, R. (1993). Fat preference and adherence to a reduced-fat diet. *American Journal of Clinical Nutrition*, 57, 373-381.

4. Rodin, J. (1978). Has the distinction between internal versus external control of feeding outlived its usefulness? In G.A. Bray (Ed.), *Recent advances in obesity research*, Vol. 2. London: Newman.

Chapter Eight

1.   Attributed to Davy Crockett.

2.   Attributed to Winston Churchill.

3.   Cormillot, A., & Fuchs, A. (1990). The possible weight. *International Journal of Obesity, 14* (Suppl.2), 10 (Abstract.)

4.   Brownell, K.D., & Wadden, T.A. (1991). The heterogeneity of obesity: Fitting treatments to individuals. *Behavior Therapy, 22,* 153-177.

5.   Jackson, A.S., & Ross, R.M. (1992). *Understanding exercise for health and fitness.* Houston, TX: CSI Software, Inc. (Table 5.1 used with permission.)

6.   Adapted from U.S. Department of Agriculture and U.S. Department of Health and Human Services. (1990). *Dietary Guidelines for Americans.* 3rd. ed. Washington, D.C.: U.S. Government Printing Office.

Appendix A

1.   Adapted from Foreyt, J.P., & Goodrick, G.K. (1991). Choosing the right weight management program. *The Weight Control Digest, 1*(6), 81-89. (Used with permission.)

APPENDIX D

SELF-EVALUATION
START OF PLAN

Eating Problems

1. How often do you overeat or binge?

    Times per week: ☐

2. How often do you eat high-fat foods
    which you knew were not
    appropriate for weight management?

    Times per week: ☐

3. How often do you eat high-sugar foods
    which you knew were not appropriate for
    weight management?

    Times per week: ☐

4. How often do you eat to soothe painful
    emotions?

    Times per week: ☐

5. How often do you feel guilt and shame for
    not controlling your eating?

    Times per week: ☐

6.   How many times have you used restrictive diets in the last 6 months?

Times: ☐

7.   How often have you used water pills or laxatives for weight management in the last 6 months?

Times: ☐

8.   How often do you skip breakfast?

Times per week: ☐

9.   How often do you eat fewer than three meals a day?

Times per week: ☐

Add up answers for an overall eating problem

score: ☐

Exercise Control

1.   How often do you exercise for at least 40 minutes?

Times per week: ☐

If less than 3, consider Chapter 6 regarding exercise motivation.

Self-Esteem

Use this scale to answer the questions below:

    1. Much less than average
    2. Less than average
    3. About average
    4. Above average
    5. Much above average

1.   Compared to the people I know, my *worth as a person* is: ☐

2. Compared to overweight people I know, my *ability to manage my weight* is: ☐

3. Compared to all people I know, my *appearance* is: ☐

4. Compared to overweight people I know, my *appearance* is: ☐

5. My *popularity among most people* is: ☐

6. My *popularity among overweight people* is: ☐

7. My ability to *control my emotions* is: ☐

8.   My *self-confidence* is: ☐

9.   My *self-control* is: ☐

Add up the answers to obtain an overall self-esteem
score: ☐

Social Connectedness

1.   How often do you *socialize*?
      Times per week: ☐

2.   How many *close friends* do you have?   ☐

3.   How many *friends can you call at 1 A.M.* to
      help you with a weight management crisis?

                                                         ☐

4.   How many *people contact you for help* with
      weight management?

                                                         ☐

5.   How often do you *get together with a group*
      to give each other support in boosting self-
      esteem and managing eating and exercise?

                                                         ☐

Add up the answers to obtain an overall social
connectedness score:

                                                         ☐

Well-Being

Use this scale to answer the questions below:

1. Very poor
2. Poor
3. Fair
4. Good
5. Excellent

My *energy* level is: ☐

My *optimism* about the future is: ☐

My career *(including housewife/mother)* is: ☐

My overall *health* is: ☐

My level of *happiness* is: ☐

Add up the answers to get on overall score for well-being: ☐

Six and 12 months from now answer this Self Evaluation Quiz again to see how much you have reduced your Eating Problem score, and improved your Exercise Control, Self-Esteem, Social Connectedness, and Well Being scores.

REPEAT SELF-EVALUATION
(6 months)

Complete this self-evaluation after doing the Plan for about 6 months. Compare your answers with your first self-evaluation.

Eating Problems

1. How often do you overeat or binge?

   Times per week: ☐

2. How often do you eat high-fat foods which you knew were not appropriate for weight management?

   Times per week: ☐

3. How often do you eat high-sugar foods which you knew were not appropriate for weight management?

   Times per week: ☐

4. How often do you eat to soothe painful emotions?

   Times per week: ☐

5. How often do you feel guilt and shame for not controlling your eating?

   Times per week: ☐

6.   How many times have you used restrictive diets in the last 6 months?

Times: ☐

7.   How often have you used water pills or laxatives for weight management in the last 6 months?

Times: ☐

8.   How often do you skip breakfast?

Times per week: ☐

9.   How often do you eat fewer than three meals a day?

Times per week: ☐

Add up answers for an overall eating problems score: ☐

Exercise Control

1.   How often do you exercise for at least 40 minutes?

Times per week: ☐

If less than 3, consider Chapter 6 regarding exercise motivation.

Self-Esteem

Use this scale to answer the questions below:

1. Much less than average
2. Less than average
3. About average
4. Above average
5. Much above average

1. Compared to the people I know, my *worth as a person* is: ☐

2. Compared to overweight people I know, my *ability to manage my weight* is: ☐

3. Compared to all people I know, my *appearance* is: ☐

4. Compared to overweight people I know, *appearance* is: ☐

5. My *popularity among most people* is: ☐

6. My *popularity among overweight people* is: ☐

7. My ability to *control my emotions* is: ☐

8. My *self-confidence* is: ☐

9. My *self-control* is: ☐

Add up the answers to obtain an overall self-esteem score: ☐

Social Connectedness

1. How often do you *socialize*?
    Times per week: ☐

2. How many *close friends* do you have? ☐

3. How many *friends can you call at 1 A.M.* to help you with a weight management crisis? ☐

4. How many *people contact you for help* with weight management? ☐

5. How often do you *get together with a group* to give each other support in boosting self-esteem and managing eating and exercise? ☐

Add up the answers to obtain an overall social connectedness score: ☐

Well-Being

Use this scale to answer the questions below:

1. Very poor
2. Poor
3. Fair
4. Good
5. Excellent

My *energy* level is: ☐

My *optimism* about the future is: ☐

My career *(including housewife/mother)* is: ☐

My overall *health* is: ☐

My level of *happiness* is: ☐

Add up the answers to get on overall score for well-being:

☐

REPEAT SELF-EVALUATION
(12 months)

Complete this self-evaluation after doing the Plan for about one year. Compare your answers with your first two self-evaluations.

Eating Problems

1. How often do you overeat or binge?

    Times per week: ☐

2. How often do you eat high-fat foods which you knew were not appropriate for weight management?

    Times per week: ☐

3. How often do you eat high-sugar foods which you knew were not appropriate for weight management?

    Times per week: ☐

4. How often do you eat to soothe painful emotions?

    Times per week: ☐

5. How often do you feel guilt and shame for not controlling your eating?

    Times per week: ☐

6. How many times have you used restrictive diets in the last 6 months?

    Times: ☐

7. How often have you used water pills or laxatives for weight management in the last 6 months?

    Times: ☐

8. How often do you skip breakfast?

    Times per week: ☐

9. How often do you eat fewer than three meals a day?

    Times per week: ☐

Add up answers for an overall eating problems score: ☐

Exercise Control

1. How often do you exercise for at least 40 minutes?

    Times per week: ☐

    If less than 3, consider Chapter 6 regarding exercise motivation.

Self-Esteem

Use this scale to answer the questions below:

1. Much less than average
2. Less than average
3. About average
4. Above average
5. Much above average

1. Compared to the people I know, my *worth as a person* is: ☐

2. Compared to overweight people I know, my *ability to manage my weight* is: ☐

3. Compared to all people I know, my *appearance* is: ☐

4. Compared to overweight people I know, *appearance* is: ☐

5. My *popularity among most people* is: ☐

6. My *popularity among overweight people* is: ☐

7. My ability to *control my emotions* is: ☐

8.   My *self-confidence* is: ☐

9.   My *self-control* is: ☐

Add up the answers to obtain an overall self-esteem
score: ☐

Social Connectedness

1.   How often do you *socialize*?
       Times per week: ☐

2.   How many *close friends* do you have?   ☐

3.   How many *friends can you call at 1 A.M.* to
       help you with a weight management crisis?
                                                    ☐

4.   How many *people contact you for help* with
       weight management?
                                                    ☐

5.   How often do you *get together with a group*
       to give each other support in boosting self-
       esteem and managing eating and exercise?
                                                    ☐

Add up the answers to obtain an overall social
connectedness score:
                                                    ☐

Well-Being

Use this scale to answer the questions below:
1. Very poor
2. Poor
3. Fair
4. Good
5. Excellent

My *energy* level is: □

My *optimism* about the future is: □

My career *(including housewife/mother)* is going: □

My overall *health* is: □

My level of *happiness* is: □

Add up the answers to get on overall score for well-being:

□

Go back and see what progress you have made in the last 12 months. Record your progress on the following page.

	START	6 MONTHS	12 MONTHS
Eating Problems			
Exercise Control			
Self-Esteem			
Social Connectedness			
Well-Being			

If you see little progress in one area study the parts of the book which concern that area. Ask your support group for additional help.

Remember:

- Stick with the Plan.

- Expect problems and setbacks.

- Always nurture.

- Never give up.

APPENDIX E

FAT GRAMS PER SERVING

Meat, fish poultry & eggs	Grams of fat/serving
Beef (3 oz trimmed of removable fat)	
corned beef	16
eye of round, roasted (select)	5
London broil, braised (choice)	12
rib, broiled (prime)	16
rib eye (Delmonico) steak, broiled (choice)	10
T-bone steak, broiled (choice)	9
top loin steak, broiled (select)	6
Luncheon meats (1 slice)	
96% Fat Free	
Turkey Pastrami	0
Oven Roasted	
Turkey Breast	0
Bologna	4
Hard Salami	3
Chicken Frank with	
Cheese	12
Seafood (3 oz cooked)	
Atlantic cod	1
haddock	1
lobster	1
salmon, pink, canned	
with bone and liquid	5
swordfish	4
tuna, canned in water	0
shrimp	1

Poultry (3 oz roasted)	**Grams of fat/serving**
chicken breast, meat with skin	7
chicken breast, meat only	3

Eggs

1 large	5
Fleischmann's Egg Beaters, 1/4 cup	0

Milk & dairy products

Milk (1 cup)

whole	8
2% fat	5
1% fat	3
skim	0
buttermilk	2

Cheese

American, 1 oz	9
cheddar, 1 oz	9
cottage cheese, 1% fat, 1 cup	2
cream cheese, 1 oz	10
mozzarella, part-skim, 1 oz	5
ricotta, part-skim, 1/2 cup	10
Swiss, 1 oz	8
Weight Watchers American Pasteurized Process Cheese Product, 1 slice	2

Yogurt	Grams of fat/serving
plain, 8 oz	7
plain nonfat 8 oz	0
plain low fat	3

Food from grains
Breads

bagel, 1	1
English muffin, 1	1
whole-wheat bread, 1 slice	1

Cereals

General Mills' Cheerios, 1 1/4 cups	2
Kellogg's Corn Flakes, 1 cup	0
Kellogg's Raisin Bran, 3/4 cup	1
Nabisco Shredded Wheat, 1 biscuit	0
Old-Fashioned Quaker Oatmeal 2/3 cup cooked	2
Quaker 100% Natural, 1/4 cup	5
Quaker Puffed Rice, 1 cup	0

Crackers

Cheese Crackers, 12	4
Graham crackers, 1 sheet	1

Other	**Grams of fat/serving**
pasta, 1 cup cooked	1
white rice, 1 cup cooked	0
pancakes, 4" plain	2
waffles, 7" plain	8
French toast, 1 slice	7

Fruits & vegetables

apple, 1 medium	1
banana, 1 medium	1
orange, 1 medium	0
raisins, 1/3 cup	0
avocado, 1/2 medium	15
broccoli, 1/2 cup cooked	0
carrot, raw, 1 medium	0
corn, canned, 1/2 cup	1
green beans, 1/2 cup cooked	0
peas, 1/2 cup cooked	0

Beans, nut & seeds

kidney beans, 1/2 cup boiled	0
lentils, 1/2 cup boiled	0
cashews, dry roasted, 1/4 cup	16
peanuts, dried, 1/4 cup	18
peanut butter, 1 tbsp	8
sesame seeds, dried, 1/4 cup	21
tahini (sesame butter), 1 tbsp	7

Spreads & oils

	Grams of fat/serving
butter, 1 tsp	4
whipped butter, 1 tsp	3
margarine, stick & tub, 1 tsp	4
diet margarine, tub, 1 tsp	2
vegetable oil, 1 tbsp	14
salad dressings, 1 tbsp	8

Soups

Campbell's Chicken Noodle, 1 cup	2
Campbell's Cream of Mushroom, 1 cup	7
Progresso Green Split Pea, 1 cup	3
Oriental Noodles & Pork Flavor, 10 oz	8

Sweets

milk chocolate with fruit & nuts, 1 oz	8
chocolate/caramel bar, 2.16 oz	14
angel food cake, 1/12 cake	0
brownie with nuts (3 x 1 x 7/8")	6
cheesecake, 1/8 cake	13
chocolate chip cookie, 2	5
Fig Newton, 1	1
apple pie, 1/8	12
banana cream pie, 1/8	12
pumpkin pie, 1/8	13
chocolate pudding, 1 cup	12

Frozen desserts **Ice cream**	**Grams of fat/serving**
vanilla fudge, 1/2 cup	8
chocolate/ chocolate chip, 1/2 cup	18

Other

Dole Fruit'N Yogurt Bar	0
Dole fruit sorbet, strawberry, 1/2 cup	0
ice cream sandwich, 3 oz bar	12
Jell-O Chocolate Pudding Pop	

Dry snack foods

microwave popcorn with butter, 4 cups popped	7
popcorn, air-popped, 1 cup, popped	0
pretzels, 1 oz	1
potato chips, 1 oz	10

SOURCE: Consumer and Food Economics Institution: *Composition of Foods-Raw, Processed, Prepared*. USDA Agricultural Handbook No. 8-1, 1976.

INDEX

accepting overweight 50
appearance 45

bearded tit mystery, the 2
beef 111
binge, from restriction 28
body dissatisfaction 46
boulder in the stream, a 6
breath holding 4

caffeine and energy cycles 85
chicken farms 111
Chinese finger puzzle, a 7
chocolate bars 110
coping with overweight,
    method one 47
    method two 49
    method three 50
    method four 51

depression and obesity 63
dieting and binging 30
dieting, failure rate 5
dieting, failure and self-blame 5
diets, causes for failure 30
drug dependency 32

eating control, loss of 30
Eating Plan, the 145
energy, recommendations 8
energy sappers 4
Energy Cycles (figure 6.1) 84
ethics and professionalism 152
evaluating weight management
    clinics quiz 154
excuse thoughts for not
    exercising 92
exercise, health benefits 89
exercise, psychological
    benefits 90
exercise, total awareness 96
exercise, disadvantages of not 90
exercise, visualization 102
exercise tips 87
exercise, stimulus control of 97
exercise, relapse 89
exercise heart rates (table 8.1) 139
exercise, cultural change 82
exercise plan 137
exercise enthusiast 81

exercise, enjoying 87

farming 81
fat gram, daily goal 141
fat and energy 113
fat cell hyperplasia 20
fat belt 16
fat cells 19
fat cell hypertrophy 20
Fat Poem, the 119
fat-to-carbohydrate ratio 35
fatigue 85
fitness clubs 97
food, environmental mismatch 4
food, as a drug 33
food environment, changing 120
food, as a drug 31
food environment 110
forest ranger's bathroom
    habits, a 7
frustrated dieters quiz, the v

getting professional help 151
goal weight 134
gradual approach 6,116
group interaction 65

happiness 50
high-fat foods, reducing desire 115
high-fat-eating, vicious cycles 114
How social support works 65
    advice 65
    control 66
    self confidence 65
    share emotions 66
    success 65
    thoughts 66

implications for the overweight 22

lookism, and the obese self 43
lookism 43
low-fat eater 110
low-fat eating, advantages 117

metabolism 19
mind control 91
mind versus body problem, the 25
models for obesity 28
monkey meat 82

monkey hunting, Peru 81

NAAFA 51
negative emotions 34
new ways of thinking 1
nonpurging bulimia 33
Nonpurging Bulimia 35

obese self, the 50,54
obese self vs. healthy self
    (table 4.1) 55
obesity, paradox 8
obesity and longevity 16
obesity, death rates 16
obesity, hereditary? 15
obesity, health risks 16
obesity, cultural differences in 16
obesity, danger 16
obesity, poverty 16
obesity, prevalence in U.S. 15
Overeaters Anonymous (OA) 72

peer support, figure 68
peer support, how to get 129
peer support 65
peers and self-esteem 66
per support, crises 69
picking your support group 70
potato chips and nutrition 111
prejudice against overweight 49
psychoactive substance
    dependance 32
Psychology of weight cycling 48
    (figure 4.1)

rain forest 81
recommended daily eating plan 145
reducing desire for
    high-fat foods 115
relapse, eating control 30
relapse 28
religion 51
resources 161
restrictive diet 29
role of genetics, adoptees 18
role of genetics, twins 17

self blame 5
self evaluation 181
self-acceptance 50
self-monitoring, food 146

self-monitoring, exercise 96
sensible eating 117
set point 20
social scrutiny 8
social support 63
social control of behavior 7
social support (figure 5.1) 68
social isolation and depression 63
social isolation and obesity 64
starting a group 131
support group, how to choose 129

The Plan 127
types of groups 71

valid excuses not to exercise 95
vanity 9,44
very low calorie diet 29
vicious cycles 85
vicious cycles related to
    high-fat eating 114
visualization, for
    couch potatoes 101
visualization, for exercisers 102

walking tips 137
weight fluctuation,
    dieter's dilemma 27
    old model 26
weight cycling, 20
tendency to stay obese 21
weight clinic, how to evaluate 154
Weight Watchers 73
willpower 64

Comments

If you have any comments about *Living Without Dieting*, please send them to the authors care of:

Harrison Publishing
P.O. Box 540515
Houston, TX 77254-0515

Ordering Information

To order additional copies of *Living Without Dieting*, please send $16.95 plus $1.50 shipping and handling to:

Harrison Publishing
P.O. Box 540515
Houston, TX 77254-0515

Don't forget to send us your address, telephone number, and drivers license number if paying by check. Texas residents please add appropriate state sales tax.

Or call:
(800) 945-6199
(713) 935-2125